PHYSICIAN ASSISTANT SCHOOL PERSONAL STATEMENT GUIDE

TIPS, TRICKS, AND TECHNIQUES TO WRITE YOUR PA SCHOOL ESSAY

SAVANNA PERRY, PA-C

PA
Platform

ABOUT THE AUTHOR

Savanna Perry, PA-C graduated from Augusta University's Physician Assistant Program in 2014. As a new grad, she created The PA Platform, a website to assist students in becoming physician assistants. After helping hundreds of students gain acceptance to PA school, Savanna is sharing her advice in this book. She currently practices in outpatient dermatology. Savanna is also the creator of The Pre-PA Club podcast.

For more information:
www.thePAplatform.com
savanna@thepaplatform.com

instagram.com/thePAplatform
youtube.com/thePAplatform
facebook.com/thePAplatform
twitter.com/thePAplatform
pinterest.com/thePAplatform

TABLE OF CONTENTS

Hey Future PA!   vii

PART 1
WHAT YOU NEED TO KNOW
1. Logistics   3
2. Reapplicants   11

PART 2
WRITING
3. Content   19
4. Mistakes   31
5. Brainstorming   41

PART 3
EDITING
6. How to Edit   49
7. Checklist   57

PART 4
ESSAY EXAMPLES
8. About this Section   63
9. Before and After   65
10. Still in Undergrad   77
11. Way Too Long   85
12. Non-Traditional Applicant   95
13. Reapplicant   103
14. Lacking Experience   111
15. GPA Issues   117
16. Patient to PA   125
17. Parent to PA Student   133
18. Resume Regurgitation   141
19. Athlete to PA   149

PART 5
BONUS SECTION

20. Experience Details   159
21. Supplemental Essays   167
22. Interview Essays   171

So What's Next?   175
Resources   179

PART 6

Notes   187

Hey Future PA!

Beyond the PA school application requirements, the essay is typically the most difficult part. Your next task is to pour your passion onto paper to show why becoming a physician assistant is your goal.

Perhaps those first words are elusive and you're struggling to begin your story. It's easy to get hung up on figuring out parts to cut out due to the character limit. No one said this was going to be easy, but after reading hundreds, maybe even thousands, of essays, I can make this mission less painful. And guess what? No essay is the same.

Everyone has a different story to tell, and your story is unique. Even without a "dramatic" event, you have pivotal moments to showcase with your uniqueness.

I can't write your essay for you or even give you a Mad Libs style template, but I can put you on a path to identifying what to include while walking you through the writing process. I've read great essays, and honestly terrible ones. Together, we will work through the process of creating an awesome and memorable essay, while avoiding detrimental mistakes.

In order to get the most benefit from this book, I recommend reading Section I and II, then completing the brainstorming worksheets. Before you begin writing your essay, review a few examples. Lastly, work on editing and polishing once you complete a draft. I look forward to writing with you! And when you need help editing, come see us at ThePAPlatform.com.

- Savanna Perry, PA-C
(Your Personal PA Coach!)

PART 1

WHAT YOU NEED TO KNOW

CHAPTER 1

LOGISTICS

While the prompt for the personal statement section can vary slightly between cycles, the change typically isn't significant. The main idea remains:

Why do you want to be a physician assistant?

Possible variations:

- Explain your motivations for wanting to become a physician assistant.
- In the space provided, write a brief statement expressing your motivation or desire to become a physician assistant.
- Discuss your motivations for becoming a physician assistant.

Do you see a theme? The majority of PA schools use a universal application service called the Centralized Application Service for Physician Assistants (CASPA) where you will directly enter your essay in text form. The character limit is **5,000 characters**, including spaces, translating to roughly one page and a paragraph single-spaced, size 12 font. Obviously, that's not a ton of space to convince someone you are the best applicant for a spot in their program, especially considering this is the most important narrative you will ever write.

In order to meet this non-negotiable requirement, you must be direct and concise. A ton of descriptors are not necessary to get your point across. Including stories is important, but the focus should remain on you. Since spaces, grammar, or punctuation cannot be sacrificed to get under the character limit, the space must be used wisely.

Once your application is submitted to CASPA, your essay **CANNOT** be edited. I want to say that again. After you have officially turned everything in, you will **NOT** have the capability to edit anything about your essay. This is important to note once you get to the editing stage, and also why your essay is not school specific. Supplemental essays allow you to expand on topics and program specific points.

In order for your essay to potentially reach the hands of an admission's committee member, the minimum requirements of each program must be met. Every school has their own process for how they choose which applications to review and how they are evaluated, but ultimately CASPA algorithms are in place to weed out applicants who don't yet check the boxes of what schools are looking for. While your essay may be amazing, if your GPA is a 2.97 and a school asks for a 3.0, it most likely won't be read. To put it simply, if your GPA, grades, experience, or test scores don't fit the minimums, your essay will never be reviewed by that particular school!

While it seems unfair, with thousands of PA school applicants, the schools need a way of separating the masses. They don't have manpower to evaluate applications of candidates who simply aren't qualified. A finished CASPA application is typically 25-35 pages long, and that's a lot to comb through! Use due diligence in making sure your application is as complete as possible before submitting.

Since schools use different processes for evaluating applications and essays, it's possible the person who reads your statement hasn't seen your entire application. Avoid reiterating everything in your app (you don't have the space), but provide enough background and detail for your reader to understand what you're referencing without searching for the information. The application may not be readily available.

WHY YOUR ESSAY IS SO IMPORTANT

On a positive note, once you meet the numerous requirements, you've cleared a large hurdle. At that point, the admissions committee is left with a smaller number of applications to evaluate and a group of people who fit their criteria, meaning your chances have improved greatly. Your essay will be the factor to set you apart. Since PA school has become so competitive, most everyone has considerable experience and an impressive resume on paper. While there will always be someone with more hours or better grades, it doesn't mean you are any less qualified or deserving.

The PA school essay is an opportunity to chronicle the unique details of your journey and express your passion for becoming a PA. I've certainly seen subpar essays result in interviews, but a thoughtful personal statement could be the difference in your acceptance. Similar to the interview process, don't focus on what you think the admissions committee wants to hear, but actually tell them about you. Your story may not be dramatic, but it's unique. The best essays I've read are ones that help me understand who the person is by the end of the essay.

THE WRITING PROCESS

Starting with a blank space is intimidating. I can only speak for myself and offer ideas in regards to the process that works best for me, and coincidentally it's why my first book (the PA School Interview Guide) took three years to complete! Don't worry about having a perfect essay from the beginning. Your first draft will definitely not be the last, and you may end up changing everything before it's considered "finished." Grammar, wording choice, and punctuation can be edited after the fact. For that matter, flow and organization can be rearranged as well. Don't let roadblocks stop you from putting initial words on paper to break the ice.

Let's review how to best use this book. This first section covers the logistical basics needed before starting on your essay with some tips for reapplicants. In Section II, we'll dive into essential content matter necessary for a strong personal statement, followed by mistakes you should avoid. Next, you'll find a chapter called "Brainstorming" consisting of worksheets to help stimulate your thoughts and organize ideas that may (or may not) make it into your essay. Think of this chpater as a guided thinking exercise.

If you aren't starting your essay in the immediate future, make a phone note or Google doc to easily store ideas from random thoughts, patient encounters, or shadowing experiences. Not everything on your list will make it into your essay, but a running list of memorable and pivotal moments can provide invaluable inspiration when the time comes.

Once you're ready to write, set yourself up for success. Choose a particular spot as a "writing area." Leave your home to go outside or visit a coffee shop, cafe, or library to remove temptations of your surroundings. Get your head in the game. Turn off the TV, close all of your browsers, and set your phone aside. If that seems daunting, set a timer to give the writing undivided attention for a set period of time. If typing your essay is a struggle, consider writing by hand, journal style, to determine if the words come easier. My writing typically starts like a journal entry from a stream of consciousness and eventually turns into a cohesive paper others can comprehend.

Another option is to speak out loud using transcription to begin your essay. The final written essay shouldn't sound like something you would speak out loud, but I find this technique helpful for writing blog posts. One suggestion is Otter, a free app that provides fairly accurate transcriptions. Think of this strategy as "interviewing" yourself to get started initially. Use the questions from Brainstorming in Chapter 5 as a starting point.

My goal is to turn this writing process from a stressful worry into an enjoyable task. In preparing for your application, the essay gives you the chance to revisit your passion and examine why you started on this path to begin with. Through all of the requirements and hurdles, it is easy to become jaded or discouraged by the long process of applying for PA school, but don't lose sight of why you committed to this journey. Try to experience the feeling of excitement you initially had for the prospects of being a PA.

WHEN SHOULD I START MY ESSAY?

Having your essay complete by the time CASPA opens in April will take a big burden off your plate to allow focus on the other parts of the application. Making a note of ideas over time, as recommended above, will make the process easier. Choose a time around December-January prior to your application cycle to really sit down and start working on your essay.

By beginning early, you'll have opportunities to step away from your writing and revisit it with a fresh mind instead of feeling rushed at the last minute. If you're planning for someone to edit your essay, that will also allow time for you to make changes and seek additional reviews.

HOW LONG WILL THIS TAKE?

That's a subjective and personal question. From literature classes throughout your education, you may have an idea of how long the writing process takes you. However, this essay is quite different because it isn't something you can just research. Your personal statement requires soul searching too, and it's so much more personal. Writing about yourself makes it more difficult, but you won't have to worry about citations.

Having dedicated writing time daily/weekly/monthly on your calendar will ensure you are allotting adequate time to focus on your essay in order to complete it by your deadline. Your timeline will depend on writing skill. Outlining and brainstorming to enter the process with organized thoughts will contribute to a more complete draft from the beginning.

SAVE YOUR WORK

Save your work!! I cannot emphasize this enough. As someone who started this book, was halfway finished, and lost all of my writing, I empathize with anyone who has experienced a technical difficulty or lost an essay.

Here are the places you do not want to save your essay: loose sheets of paper, Word document on your computer, in CASPA.

Better choices: Google Drive, Word document with an external hard drive that backs up often, possibly a note on your phone (still a little risky).

Save and back up your work often. Email your essay to yourself occasionally and save it in multiple places. Hopefully, a backup won't be needed, but do it for your own peace of mind. You won't regret it!

WHEN TO HIT SUBMIT

Speaking of deadlines, I strongly suggest setting a date to declare your essay finished. It's quite possible to continue working on your essay forever and never feel like it's complete or good enough. Look at your calendar and goals to pinpoint an ideal date you would like to have your essay finished. Early-mid April is a recommended timeline if you're shooting for submitting CASPA soon after the application cycle opens.

WRITER'S BLOCK

At some point during this process, undoubtedly, you'll feel frustrated and tempted to delete your essay and start over, or wait until next cycle. Or possibly, you won't know what to say or how to portray yourself on paper. Mixed emotions are completely normal and happen to everyone during this process.

Revisit this chapter as often as needed to refocus on what is important for your essay. If feeling stuck, try an alternate writing technique or a new setting. It's okay to take a few days off, or even a couple of weeks in order to come back to your essay with fresh eyes. If you need additional guidance and accountability to get a draft complete, visit www.thepaplatform.com/personalstatement for a free 2-week email course that will instruct you through the brainstorming phase to a complete first draft in 15-30 minutes a day.

CHAPTER 2

REAPPLICANTS

While my hope is you never find yourself in the position of reapplying, it's common. One of the main questions I receive is,

---

"Do I need to rewrite my entire personal statement?"

Valid question! Here's the thing: **Your reason for wanting to become a PA won't change significantly**, but between cycles, it's likely you have gained more experience, deepened your resolve, and matured as a person. These efforts deserve to be highlighted.

Ideally, you shouldn't submit the exact essay multiple times to the same schools through CASPA. The only exception is if you are applying to brand new schools who did not read your initial essay, but that is not typically a recommended strategy. Many schools value reapplicants. Another caveat is if you didn't meet all requirements the first time, it's unlikely they read your initial statement. In that case, you may keep the bones of the essay, but make additions to highlight your achievements since that previous submission. Some schools will keep previous application submissions and compare them, and we don't want to have you portrayed as lazy for skipping the edits.

WHAT TO CHANGE

As a second, third, or multiple time applicant, the goal is demonstrating growth to the programs you reapply to. If something didn't work the first time, there needs to be a difference in subsequent attempts. If you bake a cake that turns out dry, you wouldn't use the same recipe next time without making adjustments. This is the same concept. It's important to highlight the subjective personal changes and tangible actions you've taken to improve on any weaknesses.

If you are unsure of areas to amend for a future application cycle, my first recommendation is to consult programs you've applied to previously. Whether you received a rejection, waitlist, or no response, it's worth taking the time to request feedback. The worst thing that happens is they refuse, so it can't hurt to ask! Any information you receive will be extremely valuable to provide you with actionable steps towards making yourself a more competitive applicant. That being said, if you do ask for feedback, be prepared to follow through. For example, should a school recommend a better test score or grade, that may mean retaking courses or standardized exams. If the feedback you receive is a dealbreaker, this may be an indication it's time to move on as a specific program may not be a good fit.

In the event advice isn't offered on weak areas, evaluate yourself. Be blunt and subjective. Nitpick and look for areas that could be perceived as red flags or weaknesses by an admissions member. Ask any PAs you know to look over your application with you, as well, to get input from someone who has experience. Put yourself in the shoes of an admissions committee member and be honest about weak areas that need work. Make it your goal to provide the program with no areas for improvement.

. . .

Here are some things to consider:

- **Grades** - How are your GPAs? Are you showing an upward trend? Do they meet the minimum requirements of the schools on your list? Are they competitive for the schools you applied to? Do you have adequate grades (ideally B or higher) in required prerequisites?
- **Coursework** - Have you completed all prerequisite courses? Have you taken any recommended courses? Do you feel your transcripts demonstrate an ability to handle a PA school curriculum?
- **Experience** - Do you have a variety of experiences? Is your patient or healthcare experience hands-on? Are you getting good patient interaction and demonstrating that in your experience details? Have you filled as many categories as possible on CASPA? Does your volunteer experience show passion for your community or a certain focus? Have you shadowed broadly?
- **Testing** - (GRE, PA-CAT, MCAT) - Are your test scores competitive? Do your test scores meet the minimum requirements? Could you retake the test and potentially raise your score with additional studying?
- **Personal Statement** - That's why you're here right? More on that later.

When it comes down to what to change or include in a reapplicant essay, your reader wants to see a candidate whose passion for the field has grown despite the disappointment of an unsuccessful cycle. An applicant can demonstrate both proactive actions they've taken and personal ways they've grown through the experience. A good buzzword is "maturity." When applying to PA school as a 21-year-old, I had the opportunity to speak with a program director at an information session. I asked what they were looking for, and her response was "mature candidates." PA schools want students who understand it will be difficult and disheartening at times to attend a rigorous program and subsequently work in the medical field. The requirement of having prior experience in healthcare ensures you are ready for PA school, and you can clearly state that in your essay.

After identifying and improving weak areas, show exactly what steps you took over the year to make yourself more competitive and prepared. This may include taking classes (and performing well), gaining additional patient care hours, new volunteer experiences, improved test scores, or additional shadowing opportunities. Highlight your strengths and brag on your hard work.

HOW TO START

Having to start over may feel more daunting than the first time to sit down and restart your essay, but you're in luck! You have your initial personal statement as a starting point. Revisit your first drafts and pull out the main content points to use in your reapplicant essay. Incorporating different examples and stories will help make your essay stand apart from your first attempt.

I would encourage you to refer to the checklist in Chapter 7 and compare it with your original essay. See if you answered all of the questions and checked all of the boxes. It could be that your essay was part of the reason you didn't get the results you hoped for. If you find huge discrepancies in what you're learning in regards to what needs to be included, don't stress. Just take a breath and start from scratch. Remember, demonstrate passion and tell a story that comes from the heart. If you didn't achieve that the first time, now is your chance.

If you feel pretty good about your original essay, start with making changes to anything that wasn't achieved on the checklist. Try to sub different specifics and expand on anything that doesn't clearly express your thoughts. When it comes to adding information about personal improvements, there are two strategies. You can incorporate tidbits throughout your essay when discussing various topics like hours or grades, or save that information for closer to the end of your essay or possibly even the conclusion to make a strong finishing point. Which method you choose will depend on how your essay is set up, and you may even do a little of both.

FINAL WORDS

To be perfectly clear, I just want to reiterate that it is not recommended as a reapplicant to resubmit the exact essay to the same programs in most cases, but you don't necessarily have to start from scratch. Understandably, it stinks to make changes and spend time on it again, but if the difference is in an acceptance instead of a rejection, the time and effort will be worth it! In Chapter 13, an example of a reapplicant essay is provided to review if you get stuck.

PART 2

WRITING

CHAPTER 3

CONTENT

In regards to content, when reading a personal statement, there are a few questions I want answered. Luckily, you don't have to "choose a topic" or "pick a theme." "Why PA" is the predetermined topic. While your essay should be coherent and hopefully enjoyable to read, it isn't meant to provide entertainment value to your reader. Many try to incorporate humor, but honestly, it's not often done well. Your personality can shine through your statement to a point, but the focus should be on your story, not your jokes.

These questions will be broken down in this chapter, and with following examples you'll see them in action.

- What initially made you interested in medicine or healthcare?
- How did you find out about the PA profession? What were your first impressions?
- From that initial encounter, what happened next? Were you undecided or did you go full force ahead towards PA?
- Do you have a good understanding of the PA profession?

What have you seen while shadowing or working with PAs?
- How have you prepared for PA school?

I want you to walk me through your decision making process and the actions you've taken to get to this point. Becoming a PA isn't a decision that happens overnight. There's numerous obstacles and so much work involved, leading most people to encounter roadblocks and experience doubts along the way. Why are you one of the people who kept going?

At the end of the day, everything in your essay should directly relate back to why you are choosing this profession, and simultaneously show you are prepared to take on the challenges of PA school. Make it personal to you because anything non-specific is wasted space.

SHOW, DON'T TELL

As we delve into what to include (and not include) in your essay, consider this principle before beginning to write. The goal will be to "show" characteristics about yourself, instead of just "telling" about them. Here's an example:

- **Tell** - I have excellent time management skills.
- **Show** - While balancing a full semester and part-time job, I achieved a 4.0.

Do you see how informative the second example is? By carefully using specific word choices to highlight your passion or strengths rather than telling about them, the better the essay overall. Include in depth information and your essay will be more engaging. The main focus should be to incorporate a wide variety of subtle quality traits without just stating the obvious. In the "Brainstorming" chapter, you'll have the opportunity to list what makes a successful PA. These adjectives are the pillars to begin thinking about now.

This concept translates to your experiences as well. Recounting a patient story or interaction with a PA will be more memorable than just stating it happened. Here is an example:

- **Tell** - While shadowing Megan, I noticed she spent a lot of time with patients. I want to be a PA because they can prescribe medications.
- **Show** - I followed Megan into the patient's room and noticed how she developed a rapport by asking about the patient's family. Then, she wrote out instructions after prescribing a new medication to aid the patient in understanding her treatment plan.

This example turns a simple statement into a short story. There is a fine line between having an engaging essay and being "over the top." It doesn't take dramatics to make a point. While you may encounter faculty who get roped into a catchy story, eventually anything farfetched gets old after hundreds of essays, so use descriptors appropriately. If your essay doesn't incorporate adjectives and imagery, it's likely to err on the boring side. As a rule of thumb, try to use only one descriptive word per example in your essay. This technique will save on characters and allow for more meaningful content in your essay, like this:

- **Multiple descriptors** - During my time with Megan, she showed kindness and compassion with patients.
- **One descriptor** - During my time with Megan, she was compassionate with patients.

Don't stress too much about writing techniques until you have decided on a good footprint. Revisit these principles to make your essay interesting and memorable. While stories may be from your healthcare experience, it's okay to include ones from everyday life as well. If you do include a story involving a patient, change identifying information to avoid HIPAA violations. Should you decide to address a personal/family/work medical issue, be cognizant that your audience is made up of medical people! I've read essays that vaguely allude to a medical problem, however specifics are preferable. Perhaps you are uncomfortable giving a name to a condition or diagnosis, and in that case consider leaving this particular scenario out of your essay. As the reader with a medical education, omitting a diagnosis comes off strange and leaves the reader with doubt surrounding the situation.

Set the scene as quickly as possible, identify your role, and establish your point. If a detail isn't essential to the meaning of the story or the end result, take it out. Even if it's an eloquent description, you'll likely need that space elsewhere. Most importantly, any example used must have a main point. Whether it's a lesson you learned, an illustration about your personality, or a direct influence on you to choose PA, you're not just telling a story to tell it. Space is limited, and your reader doesn't have time for frivolities. Use supplemental essays to expand on stories you aren't able to fully tell in your personal statement.

USING PERSONAL INFORMATION

If I've said it once, I've said it a million times - the more personal you can be throughout this process, the better. Your essay is a means to highlight your personality, background, and attributes. You can't solely rely on your experience and accolades to carry you. PA schools are looking for a well-rounded, interesting person as an applicant and potential student. They want to see someone with unique interests outside of medicine. The essay offers an opportunity to jump off the paper and become someone they are excited to meet at an interview. Keep it professional, but personable. Sell yourself to your reader!

Don't confuse being open with imposing drama in your essay.

That's not necessarily the best way to accomplish this task. Just tell your story directly. Some of the best essays I've read are not ones with a huge "aha" moment, but ones I can honestly say, "I feel like I know this person well, and I believe they are ready for PA school" by the end. Without the distraction of an intense scenario, it's easier to focus on the core reasons the applicant is choosing to become a PA.

Although sharing personal information can be difficult, the more vulnerable you're willing to get, the better (in most cases). We've been patients or watched friends or family become patients at some point. Sharing how those experiences were inspiring, discouraging, or intriguing injects honesty into your writing. Throughout life, you may be in awe with a growing interest in medicine, comforted by a caring provider, or interacting with a healthcare professional who becomes a role model. These situations are important to include if they've made an impact on you.

During an interview with Allan Platt, admissions director at Emory University, we discussed reading an essay about a sick grandparent as someone's first introduction to the PA profession, and how all they could think about was becoming a PA. He emphasized the focus of an experience should be on compassion for the family member and not on personal goals. It's possible to tactfully include information about the impact of a personal health situation, while still showing concern for a family member. Mr. Platt's interview is available on The Pre-PA Club podcast.

When addressing a family member, patient, or PA, use names. It gives your essay a more personal feel and helps with following the story. If someone has a very long name, feel free to shorten or change for HIPAA purposes and alter any identifying information.

While I've stated the need to be personal, there are often questions about how personal. Here is what your personal statement is not - your plan to fix healthcare, an attempt to gain sympathy, a declaration of the injustices you've faced. There are a few controversial topics that don't have a place in your essay, and politics is the main one. I haven't read an essay that makes a good case for how discussing personal values relates directly to becoming a PA, whereas a non-judgmental attitude is an integral part of working in medicine. In regards to personal medical issues, mental health is the area that comes up most frequently. Share as much as you feel comfortable, if it is relevant to you becoming a PA. If you're unsure about a topic, ask yourself whether the information being shared could raise doubts about your ability to successfully finish PA school. In most cases, it comes down to how an issue is presented, and focusing on growth and positivity are key.

PIVOTAL MOMENTS

Referring back to the initial questions at the beginning of this chapter, consider the pivotal moments along your journey. What stands out when you consider everything you've done so far? Think through significant situations that shine during your PA journey. What influencers have helped you reach this goal or held you back? Take advantage of this opportunity to get personal with your reader by sharing your story.

Let's begin with how you discovered an interest in medicine. Where exactly should you start and how far back should you go? Ultimately, it's up to you. Many people state their initial interest in medicine originated in childhood with a personal illness or family illness. That circumstance is common and makes sense. Other applicants recall a meaningful event making them desire more knowledge about medicine. If your healthcare interest was found later in life, explain what shifted or changed to inspire you.

Once your motivation is understood, include how you found out about the PA profession. The Physician Assistant Education Association (PAEA) 2020 Student Report lists previous health care experience, other PA acquaintance, PA who treated me/my family, or family member as the most common sources of influence in making a decision towards becoming a PA. According to the same report, the majority of people decide to become a PA either during the first two years of college, during the second two years of college, or after receiving a Bachelor's degree. The main takeaway from this data is most people aren't entering college wanting to be PAs. It's considered a newer profession with little common knowledge in the general population, unlike nursing or medical school.

If this story sounds familiar, that's completely okay. From working with applicants, the majority consider medical school in some capacity, or nursing as well. This was the case for me. I learned about the PA profession during high school, but I didn't have a personal encounter until shadowing my freshman year in college. That experience solidified my decision to pursue PA because until that point, I was pre-med. Admissions committees realize this too. You won't be dinged for altering a plan that wasn't originally directed toward PA school. We will look directly at how you made that decision.

Side note - No worries if you don't have a lightbulb origin story or a dramatic event confirming you should pursue healthcare or become a PA. Honesty, genuine reasons, and speaking from passion stands out beyond a cool story. Your story and uniqueness is not insignificant. Everyone is different with their own motivations for pursuing medicine and becoming a PA. As a reminder, stay away from the dramatic story. Avoid personal doubts that prevent you from writing your best essay with unfounded comparisons of how much better someone else's may be.

From there, we navigate to the point of "why PA?" fairly quickly. This is the meat of your essay and your moment to prove yourself to your reader. The 2020 PAEA Student Report includes the main reasons matriculating students chose to become PAs. Students self-reported and could choose multiple options. Here are the results with greater than 50% response rate:

- Desire to care for patients
- Work-life balance
- **Mobility within PA specialties**
- Financial Stability
- Excitement of health care
- **Length of education**
- A "calling" to the health care profession

While many of these themes apply to other medical professions, I've highlighted the PA specific ones. You need to go beyond these buzzwords to characterize the daily roles and responsibilities as the most important aspects and delineate how you will do those things specifically as a PA. If the information in your essay could be applied to any other healthcare profession and still make sense, it's too general.

The next question in the student survey asked why students chose PA over other health professions for their careers. The response "PA profession was a better fit for my personality" won by a landslide. To show how PA is a better fit, make your explanation show your personality. Complete confidence in your decision to become a PA should be passionately stated and abundantly apparent to the reader. Using stories from personal experiences will be the most effective way to incorporate this information. If addressing volunteer work or patient care experience, I don't just want to hear about a task, but details of why and the impact, which returns to the "show, don't tell" principle.

Include real encounters with patients and PAs to illustrate your understanding of the PA profession. Sharing your role in personal stories will further demonstrate personality characteristics and strengths you will bring to a PA program. Use this moment to brag on yourself! In general, people struggle with talking about themselves, but in this setting, it's not a choice. A busy CASPA application with various entries and dates doesn't always let your hard work shine. If you worked full-time while going to school or juggled college level sports with a full course load, these are things you may want to mention.

When using stories, keep the focus on you - your role, your lessons, and how a particular experience impacted your path to becoming a PA. Avoid shifting focus onto the subject of your example because you don't have space to waste talking about other people. Uncle George sounds like a great guy, but I should learn more about you than him. A large amount of material I remove when editing is insignificant details about others. Choose examples based on the filter of how it relates to you becoming a PA.

While detailing these points, keep your information in chronological order when possible. Your timeline should be simple to follow with cues provided to help your reader understand when events are occurring. For additional support with figuring out flow, check out Chapter 6 for Editing advice.

One final note, maintain honesty in your essay. Showing your genuine self cannot be faked. Don't attempt to stretch the truth or add a little drama in order to gain sympathy. If something in your essay doesn't match up with your application or seems questionable, the reader could write you off and set your application aside. Trust me, they've heard it all!

INTRODUCTION

There are multiple ways to grab your reader's attention. We've been taught to have a "hook" throughout English classes, but it isn't always necessary to start with a crazy story, and honestly, those types of intros get a bit old. They sometimes feel forced if too dramatic, and require a stretch of imagination to connect it to your "why PA?" If you have an interesting anecdote connected to the prompt, go for it. Otherwise, just jump into your story. I do recommend using a story perspective, while keeping the timeline of your overall journey in mind to help with flow.

Personally, I don't plan my introduction until the writing is pretty much done because it can change. Staring at a blank piece of paper is intimidating, so initially your goal is to get some words on the paper. In our "Essay Examples" section, you're provided with multiple ways to begin your essay, but don't be tempted to copy these directly. Use information gathered in the Brainstorming section to provide an idea of what will be most impactful for your first impression.

CONCLUSION

You need a conclusion! This paragraph should be a strong, separate statement (it can be short) summing everything up, emphasizing your strengths, and showing why you are the BEST person for a spot in PA school. Utilize your last words as an attempt to convince your reader you are ready to take the next step towards becoming a PA. At some point in your essay, address your academic strength to reassure the reader you are ready to be successful as a PA student. If you haven't already demonstrated scholar, the conclusion is a great place.

There's no need to address your reader directly in your conclusion or any part of your essay. Avoid a general phrase like "Thank you for your consideration" as it just takes up space. I encourage ending dynamically with a confident statement about you being a PA. Reference the good (and bad) conclusion examples in Section IV.

ACCEPTABLE TERMINOLOGY

There are a few small caveats in the terminology surrounding the PA profession. Don't forget your audience - academic physician assistants. One of your goals is demonstrating a full understanding of the PA profession. Visit the AAPA.org website to verify terminology and mirror the wording used on program websites throughout the application.

For example, "Advanced Practice Provider (APP)" has replaced "mid-level" in reference to PAs or NPs. Mid-level indicates different levels of care and isn't a great description of how PAs practice.

Another example is in the discussion of working as part of a healthcare team. "Collaborating physician" is generally more acceptable than "supervising physician" for discussion of the teamwork relationship between a PA and the doctor they work with (not under). There's a progressive movement for PAs to be regarded as an integral part of the healthcare team, which your wording can reflect.

Let's discuss abbreviations, which are acceptable and space-saving, if done correctly. After the first time you write out "physician assistant (PA)," you may use the PA abbreviation throughout the rest of your essay. Here are the correct ways to refer to PAs:

- Physician assistant (PA) - I shadowed a physician assistant (PA) for the first time.
- Physician assistant's (PA's) - I enjoyed the physician assistant's (PA's) demeanor.
- Physician assistants (PAs) - I shadowed all of the physician assistants (PAs) in the office.

This goes for anything you want to shorten. First time use should be written out completely, followed by the abbreviation, with subsequent use of just the abbreviation in the remainder of your essay. This is particularly important if it is not a well known abbreviation, but standard practice for a formal essay.

ADDRESSING RED FLAGS

A rule of thumb when deciding if application issues need to be addressed in your essay comes down to a single question - *Would [insert issue] potentially prevent me from getting an interview?* If the answer is yes, include it. If not, use your supplemental essays or interviews as an opportunity to address the issue.

Some "red flags" I get questions about include low grades/GPAs/test scores, lack of experience, misdemeanors, and gaps in education or work. Be assured if you meet the requirements a program is asking for, you are automatically a competitive applicant! There's no place in your application for self-degradation.

When it comes to grades, I consider "low" as C or below, but use discernment in deciding whether to include an explanation of every grade. A few blips, with an overall upward trend, likely won't have much effect on your potential of securing an interview. If you had significant struggles with a certain course or semester, briefly include a statement about efforts you made and beneficial lessons. Typically, a gap in education or experience won't need an explanation unless there are particular circumstances you would like to include. Specific examples are detailed in the Essay Examples section.

If you lack patient care, volunteering, or shadowing hours, please don't state that directly. Focus on what you DO have and what you've learned following those experiences. Your experiences have already been vetted and approved if your essay is being read.

You can skip discussing misdemeanors or other legal issues in your essay because there is a separate section on the application to include this information. You aren't allowed an abundance of space to explain, but it should be sufficient for making your case outside of the personal statement. Supplemental applications may also provide another space to expand on previous mishaps.

If you identify a questionable aspect on your application and decide to address it, be direct, to the point, and keep it concise. Ideally, start with the positive and save the last third of your essay to address areas of needed improvement. Don't devote a ton of space to negative aspects and avoid the appearance of making any type of excuse. 1-3 sentences should suffice to state the issue, give a brief explanation of why, and most importantly, show how you've grown and learned from that situation. The next chapter on Mistakes will expand on what NOT to do in your essay, and then we'll start writing!

CHAPTER 4

MISTAKES

Now that we've discussed what to include, it's important to address common mistakes - aka things not to do in your essay. Keep these suggestions in mind while writing in order to make the final editing steps easier. The information I'm including is not meant to shake your confidence, but to provide beneficial feedback based upon what I've seen work (and not work). These insights come from applications and discussions with various faculty and admissions directors.

As an editor, I see these repeatedly, so don't feel discouraged if you notice your essay includes similar mistakes. While reading this chapter, you may think I'm exaggerating while mentioning these issues, but you would be surprised. The Essay Examples in Section IV will allow you to identify mistakes in real essays.

PLAGIARISM

Don't copy your essay. Don't use a template. Do use your own words and thoughts. These are things I shouldn't have to say, but stress makes people do crazy things. Ethical integrity is a standard at all PA programs.

APPLICATION REGURGITATION

You can and should touch on experiences, but avoid repeating all of the information directly from your resume. If you include a specific experience, expand on what you actually learned and took away from those hours instead of simply repeating what your role was. Make a strong case for why each activity has influenced your decision to become a PA. The example in Chapter 18 demonstrates how listing everything straight from your application doesn't make for a dynamic essay.

Here is an example of how NOT to include a discussion of an experience:

I worked as a certified nursing assistant (CNA) at Aiken Regional Hospital for four years. It was a rewarding direct patient care experience. I worked with PAs and saw them take care of patients.

While your experience is important and shouldn't be discounted, what truly matters is your future intentions as you move forward into PA school and your profession as a PA. Pull out a patient story from that experience to expand on instead of only providing superficial information.

"PHYSICIAN'S ASSISTANT"

As a future PA, it's imperative to know the name of your career, and while it could potentially change, right now it is physician assistant. NO apostrophe "s." That is a huge red flag. Am I personally offended when someone gets it wrong? Not at all, but think about your audience of academic PAs. (This goes for interviews too.)

FORGETTING TO EDIT

Don't skip Chapter 6! By all means, run a spell check. After editing and polishing your essay until it is as close to perfect as possible, have someone else edit it further.

GETTING OFF TOPIC

Straying from the prompt happens in a variation of ways - telling a story that takes up your entire essay, hating on one of the many flaws in healthcare systems, or reiterating your application. When you read back through your essay, everything included needs to directly relate to why you want to be a PA. If it doesn't answer that question, delete it. This is not an essay about how you would fix the healthcare system or your goals to build a clinic and help overseas. Those are magnificent ambitions, and you may get a chance to expand in supplementals, however stay on track for your main personal statement.

TRYING TO USE THEMES

Your essay already has a theme - "Why PA." Comparing the PA profession to playing soccer or picking fruit is a common tactic, but it often doesn't work and inevitably takes up valuable space. The best essays I've read just jump right into discussing medicine, they address the prompt from the very beginning and begin their discussion around the PA profession early. Your reader is reviewing hundreds or thousands of essays, don't make them think too hard to figure you out by trying to follow a theme. Using repetitive phrases to prove a point also falls under this category. I would rather see a great transition than wasted space with the same quote or sentence throughout your essay.

VERB TENSE

I'm getting nit-picky, but this applies to experience details also. Use consistent and appropriate verb tense. Go back to English class for a minute. If you are currently working in a position, use present tense - "I take vital signs and history." If you have left a job, use past tense - "I took vital signs and history." Switching between the two is confusing.

IGNORING ACADEMIC STRENGTHS

You're currently applying for a position as a PA student, not yet as a PA. If you're at the point of applying, you must feel confident in your academic capabilities, so it's up to you to convince your reader of that. If you don't feel confident, but you meet the requirements, you're still a competitive applicant. Talk up your strengths! While this doesn't have to take up a huge portion of your essay, it should be addressed in at least 1-2 sentences.

PUTTING DOWN OTHER PROFESSIONS

In regards to being positive, we all know PAs are awesome, but we are NOT any better than other members of the healthcare team. There are great PAs and bad PAs, the same way as there are great doctors and bad doctors. Avoid comparison in this manner, as much as possible, even if you were personally involved in a situation where you feel the PA was "right" or "better" than the doctor. You can emphasize the PA's performance without throwing anyone else under the bus. The same goes for nurses, nurse practitioners, or any healthcare professional. PAs are expected to be team players and you need to portray that attitude throughout your essay.

HATING ON HEALTHCARE

If you've gained patient care experience, you are likely aware there are a lot of issues in healthcare: insurance problems, unethical situations, lack of access, etc. One of the reasons PA schools require direct experience is to confirm you can handle that aspect of working in medicine, but be cautious to avoid negativity in your essay. Focus on the positives unless you're asked directly about an issue on supplemental essays. Instigating a discussion on the downfall of the US healthcare system can be a huge rabbit hole and take up too much of your essay.

GETTING POLITICAL

Politics and controversial topics were briefly addressed in the last chapter, but to reiterate, your personal statement isn't the place for stating your opinions or positions on these matters. Avoid polarizing views that may turn your reader off from thinking you can provide non-biased care unless directly asked in a prompt.

NEVER SAYING PHYSICIAN ASSISTANT

It would be an exaggeration to say I've seen essays that NEVER say "physician assistant," but I've certainly seen multiple that only mention PA in the conclusion paragraph. Yikes! Going back to what the prompt is about, PA needs to be directly discussed early in your essay, preferably by the 2nd or 3rd paragraph.

Ideally, you should be making connections to yourself as a PA throughout your essay. Avoid general phrases, such as "When I'm a healthcare professional, XYZ." No! You are trying to become a PA. Own that with confidence and convince your reader to recognize you in that role by saying "When I'm a PA!"

LISTS

Writing a formal essay means lists are not invited to the party. Here's a list of the lists you don't need to include in your essay:

- Everything you know about the PA profession that could also be based on a Google definition
- An excessive use of descriptors about the same subject
- An account of experience listing every job responsibility
- Every class you completed during or after undergrad

POINTING OUT WEAKNESSES

Positivity and strengths take you further, and make for a more enjoyable read, versus dwelling on weaknesses. Everyone can recognize areas of deficiency in their application, and there's no such thing as a perfect application. Hopefully, knowing you aren't alone will give additional confidence in emphasizing strengths you can bring to the program making you a valuable classmate and future colleague.

STRETCHING THE TRUTH

Honesty was mentioned in the previous chapter, but even stretching or manipulating the truth is unwise. Be ready for questions on anything you include in your essay at an interview and being called out for anything questionable. The majority of your application is based on the honor system, but any wild claims may be followed up with research or confrontation.

@*#& AND OTHER 4 LETTER WORDS

Did I ever think I would need to caution against the use of curse words in a graduate school essay? Definitely not! Is this based on an actual personal statement intro that incorporated cuss words as part of a patient quote? Yes it is! Guys, there is no place for this in your essay. Please refrain from profanity.

OUT OF SCOPE

I know the mission trip you took to the Philippines was an absolutely amazing experience and you saw a ton of cool stuff. While there, the doctor you shadowed even let you suture and perform circumcisions! Surely that will make you stand out, right?

You're correct, but not in the way you hope. Ethics are a hot topic in PA school, and medicine in general. There is a lot of buzz around "scope of practice," especially surrounding international scenarios. This means doing only what's in your job description even in a different location or country. If you are working as a CNA, MA, EMT, or even a registered nurse in America, you likely aren't suturing or performing circumcisions. It's out of your scope. When traveling to another country, you're expected to practice in the same scope as in the US, based on your education and certifications. As a PA, it's the same for me. When I went to Kenya, I still had a collaborating physician available. Be cautious with choosing to share these types of experiences in your essay in order to prevent schools from doubting your ethics before ever meeting you. (PS - This example comes from a real applicant.)

NOT BEING SPECIFIC ENOUGH

As you review your essay, if something is included that looks as if it could be found and written with a simple Google search, it isn't specific enough. This common mistake is seen mainly in discussions of what being a PA entails or what makes it appealing. Physician assistant is consistently ranked as one of the top professions in the US, and there are tons of perks like lateral mobility, job flexibility, a strong salary to cost ratio, and plenty of demand. This sounds good, but what about the actual job? The daily grind of what PAs do everyday? That is what's important! Avoid excess focus on popular phrases, such as "lateral mobility" or "work life balance." Those are concepts you can pursue in any profession and plenty of PAs work more than their physician counterparts. Schools are hoping to admit applicants who love the profession and the job of being a PA.

The other mistake in this regard is omitting essential information about your role when telling a story. Your reader may not have your application immediately in front of them to refer to. The details of your role will remain a mystery if you say "While I was working at the hospital I saw PAs." Adding a simple comment helps, like "While I was working at the hospital **as a CNA** I saw PAs." Context is key in providing enough information to express your story clearly. If you're referring to someone by a name, you need to also include the title or connection to avoid confusion.

BEING TOO SPECIFIC

To continue, it is also possible to be too specific. Although I see this less often, I more often request more details in edits. From the previous example, it would be a little overkill and unnecessary to say "While I was working at East Regional Community Hospital as a CNA in the neurology department, I saw neurology PAs." Name-dropping a facility usually doesn't matter. It's not a bad idea to include some information about the types of populations you've been exposed to, but avoid redundancy.

LETTING DRAMA TAKE THE STAGE

For some reason, most applicants feel the need to have a dramatic story at some point in their essay. I've heard it all - a dark and stormy night, the random person just fell out and you were the only one there, you urgently needed [insert body part] surgery. Oftentimes these stories seem like stark exaggerations with ultimately nothing to do with the writer's intentions of becoming a PA. I want to know your story, but being over the top in descriptions comes off as a desperate cry for material. Skip the dramatic approach and instead, use simple storytelling, descriptive language, and facts to depict passion for entering the PA profession.

ALL ABOUT SALLY

One of the most common mistakes is the use of stories without a clear purpose. When I finish reading about your patient, Sally, I should know more about your involvement and what you achieved than what was wrong with her. While I hope the scenario has a favorable outcome, what happened to the patient is honestly not important in the grand scheme of why you aspire to become a PA. In the essay examples, you'll ascertain how to effectively use stories to emphasize your point. Try to identify the irrelevant ones as well.

I occasionally get asked about "name-dropping" prestigious doctors or supervisors. I don't typically recommend this technique. People who may be well-known in your area usually lack widespread familiarity. Consider asking for a letter of recommendation from those individuals, particularly with a connection to a program.

MENTIONING SPECIFIC PROGRAMS

The majority of PA programs use the universal CASPA application, which means if you apply to multiple programs you submit ONE essay that goes to ALL programs. Simply put, don't talk about how much you love Duke's curriculum and send it to Yale. Whoops! Schools are aware you're likely applying to multiple places, but don't need it rubbed in their faces. Every program wants to feel they are number one on your list, and supplemental essays will most likely present an opportunity to provide school-specific information.

On the flip side, if you are applying to a non-CASPA school with a separate personal essay, working on supplemental essays, or only applying to one school, be school-specific. Keep the prompt in mind of "Why PA?" and don't get too far off track talking about the program, but you can cater your essay to their specific needs. Do your research on the program's website, review the mission statement, and identify the types of students they generally tend to accept.

QUOTES, DIALOGUE, AND CLICHÉS

"Nobody cares how much you know until they know how much you care."
   -Theodore Roosevelt

I'm not sure how many times I've seen that one, but it's a lot! I can't think of a situation when I've recommended leaving a quote in an essay. They come off as cliché and an easy way out to fill space. I doubt most people can truly say there is a quote they "live by" or think about that much. Maybe a song lyric, but don't use those either. Scripture may play a large role in your life, but I would also caution against including a verse in your essay.

Dialogue between people is also rarely done well. Most often, it just breaks the flow and becomes hard to follow. Tell the story in a different way and avoid dialogue if possible.

Quotes fall into the cliché category, but it also includes common sayings or thoughts that make you want to roll your eyes. For example, "I want to help people." Don't we all? If that's your motivation, that's wonderful, but go beyond into telling how you've already helped people and plan on continuing as a PA student and PA.

Time to start writing! Are you ready?

CHAPTER 5

BRAINSTORMING

It's time to put ideas on paper. The previous chapters should have you in the right mindset, but if you're staring at a blank sheet of white paper, don't fret, writer's block is normal. Use these worksheets to begin the process of organizing your thoughts for your personal statement. Starting is the hardest part, therefore treat these prompts as mini journal entries. Don't think about writing in regards to your essay, but just get some ideas on paper. Sentences or bullet points are perfectly fine for this exercise. No pressure here.

I recommend designating a specific period of time to work on this assignment. Set 30-60 minutes on a timer and tune the rest of the world out. Put your phone on "do not disturb" and avoid checking email or notifications. Turn the TV off and keep distractions away to focus on soul searching for the next few questions in this chapter. Be honest and take time to reflect on past experiences and what has brought you to this point. If you get stuck on one question, skip it and come back to it later. Tap into the passion that initially inspired you to pursue the PA profession and start getting excited about the next steps.

. . .

What are the initial "pivotal moments" that come to mind?

What initially made you interested in medicine or healthcare?

How did you learn about physician assistants?

. . .

How did you feel after that initial encounter with PAs? What were your thoughts?

What is appealing to you about becoming a PA? List the aspects of the profession you are most excited about.

. . .

Did you consider other medical professions? What made those more or less appealing than PA? Did this play a major role in your story?

What are memorable experiences you had while shadowing or working with PAs?

Do you have a strong understanding of the PA profession? How would you define a PA's job?

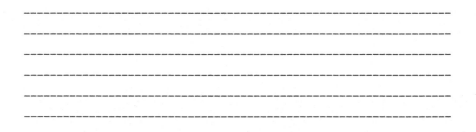

. . .

List the qualities that make a successful PA.

How have you prepared to be successful as a PA student? How will
that translate into success as a PA?

What lessons from patient care/healthcare experiences stand out?

. . .

What lessons have you learned from volunteering?

Are there any discrepancies on your application that you need to address?

What are your goals as a PA?

PART 3

EDITING

CHAPTER 6

HOW TO EDIT

When editing your essay, consider three main components:

- Content - Are you answering the essential questions?
- Grammar, spelling, and punctuation
- Flow - Does your essay make sense? Is it organized chronologically without creating confusion?

Although the end goal is not necessarily to produce an amazing piece of literature, your essay should be enjoyable to read and easy to follow. At a graduate level program, schools want to see proper and accurate language skills. Although you may never write another essay after PA school, you will frequently write patient notes. Providers need to understand with clarity what you're saying, and a confusing essay may raise red flags about your ability to communicate.

Let's break down editing steps and resources to get you going. This process may feel overwhelming, especially if you are over on characters or feeling unconfident in your essay. Here are some steps to make the process easier. While you may not utilize all of them, use these if you're feeling stuck.

1. **Set a deadline.** Decide when you want your personal statement to be considered complete, and mark the date on a calendar. Ask a friend, relative, or co-worker to hold you accountable and post the date in a prominent location. There will come a point in this editing process where you'll want to continue rechecking everything, but eventually, it just has to be done!

2. **Run spell check.** You would think everyone does this step, but after editing many essays - they don't. The spell check in Word or Google docs is a good place to start. Grammarly is an online service that is like a spell check on steroids. There's a free option, so take advantage!

3. **Read your essay out loud as you record yourself.** Yes, this will feel awkward, but do it anyway. Hearing your essay will help you identify strange wording or flow issues that need resolved.

4. **Print out your essay and edit it by hand.** Grab a highlighter or colored pen to physically mark your essay. Staring at a computer screen for hours can make the words run together. Switch it up for the sake of your eyes and see if there's anything you missed.

5. **Read through multiple times focusing on one specific thing at a time** - spelling, punctuation, grammar, and flow. Then consider each content question from chapter 3.

6. **Refer to the checklist in chapter 7.** Can you confidently answer all questions with a yes? If not, fix the needed changes and restart this process.

7. **Outside opinions.** Time to ask for help. (More on that topic later in this chapter.)

8. Repeat any of the above steps as needed until you feel confident in your essay, and **put it away until submission time**!

5,000 CHARACTERS

Through your editing, keep the goal of <5,000 characters (including spaces) in mind. It's not a suggestion, but a non-negotiable rule. Through editing, I've seen some creative attempts to cut down on space. My favorites were deleting all spaces between sentences and removing the majority of punctuation. Please refrain from either option as it makes the essay extremely difficult to read.

If you find yourself over the character limit, no doubt you can make minor changes to shorten your essay, leading to a better result. Remember our goal - direct and concise. Go through your essay and look to see if you can make any of these changes:

- **Abbreviations**. Done correctly, there is no reason to write out "physician assistant" 20 times. Look for other common phrases to shorten.
- **Repetition**. This refers to words, ideas, points, descriptions, facts, etc. Examples in the next section provide instances where the content can be simplified to save on characters.
- **Pick one.** When using descriptions, be choosy. Describing a PA as "kind and compassionate" takes up much more space than just saying "kind." Comb your essay for lists or anything connected with the word "and" to see where you can cut back.
- **4 letter words.** These words should never make it into your essay - that, very, really, have (to), (be) able (to), pretty, probably. Focus on active verbiage. Ex - **I was able to shadow Joe** vs **I shadowed Joe**.
- **Implied information.** This is best shown with an example. **I think I will be a great PA** vs **I will be a great PA**. The "I think" part is implied so take it out.

CONTENT

Content is the most important part of your essay so this could take a while. At the end of your essay, these simple questions need to be answered:

- Would I want this person taking care of me/my family?
- Do I have a complete picture of who this person is?
- Would I want to be a classmate to this person?
- Does this person fully understand the role of a PA?
- Can I confidently say this person is committed to becoming a PA?

Reread your essay through the lens of each prompt. Remember the main question of, "Why PA?" Everything included in your essay should ultimately relate back to answering this question directly or lead to the prompt in some way. If a story, detail, or example isn't related, it likely doesn't belong in your personal statement. It isn't bad information, but when space is limited, omit unrelated information. Supplemental applications will afford opportunities to expand, which is detailed at the end of the book.

Reread your essay again through the eyes of an admissions director. Is anything confusing? Hard to follow? Are there red flags? Your reader is sifting through thousands of essays. They need you to get to the point while keeping their attention. The last thing the reader wants to do is go search for information in your application.

To determine whether material should be included, ask these questions:

- What's the purpose?
- What's the impact?
- Why does this matter?

Remove holes from your story, as the focus remains on you. Evaluate the stories and examples in search of the main character. It should be you! The reader is seeking what an experience says about you rather than someone else in the scenario.

GRAMMAR, SPELLING, AND PUNCTUATION

I'm not going to give a complete grammar lesson here, but I will point out common mistakes. This is where it's imperative to double and triple check for small things you may have missed. Are a few small mistakes deal breakers? Not necessarily, but they are often easily avoidable.

For abbreviations, the first time you use a phrase, it should be spelled out completely followed by the abbreviation in parentheses. However, if you don't use that phrase/abbreviation in the essay again, don't include it as a reference. The essay examples will show you the correct method.

Pay attention to how you word and format your sentences. Avoid run-ons, sentence fragments, and be direct. Have someone read your essay to help decipher if sentence structure is an issue.

Check for spelling (actually run spell check), punctuation, and capitalization. If you decide to capitalize a phrase, such as Physician Assistant, keep it consistent throughout your personal statement. It's not necessarily wrong, but physician assistant does not typically need capitalized unless you're using it in a title.

FORMATTING TIPS

Tabs don't transfer to CASPA, meaning you won't have traditional paragraph breaks, however you still need to break up your text. It's extremely hard to read an entire block of words. Accomplish this by adding a double Enter/Return in between paragraphs.

Also, special characters, italics, bold, strikethrough, underline are all formatting techniques that don't transfer to CASPA. I've seen all of these submitted in essays for editing, but you don't want anything funky to happen when you try to submit your application.

FLOW

After content, I personally think flow is the next most important aspect of a personal statement. A confusing timeline in an essay can overshadow great information or writing. When it feels random and all over the place, it's more difficult to follow. Make reading your essay easy and enjoyable.

Presenting your information in chronological order is typically best. Your reader may not have your complete application while reading your essay. Without adequate details, it is difficult to figure out if you're referring to a certain experience. Adding just a little bit of context with dates and timing is very helpful. Pay attention to techniques in the essay examples.

In addition to a solid timeline, use transitions between topics. Abruptly jumping from subject to subject feels a little strange. As a reader, this writing style makes me wonder how your experiences are connected. These issues are also highlighted in the next section.

ASKING FOR HELP

You definitely need other eyes on your essay. Not only for their opinions, but you'll go crazy trying to edit it yourself.

The easiest option is family, friends, or co-workers. These people know you best and can determine if your essay sounds personally authentic, which is important feedback. The downside is their lack of knowledge about what PA school applications should look like. Your mom is inclined to tell you, "Honey, it sounds great!" That's not super helpful. You may also consider using a stranger for an objective view, but take their familiarity with PA school admissions processes into account. If someone does not know you personally, they can gauge how much personality is incorporated without a biased view.

Ideally, have a PA edit your essay, or at least read it for additional feedback. Perhaps someone you work with or shadowed, keeping in mind that just because someone is a PA, it doesn't mean they are in tune with school requirements. While many PAs go through the application process and never look back or stay current with changes, they can tell if your interpretation of the PA profession is correct.

Look into resources at your school if you are enrolled. Ask an advisor or career center counselor if they have workshops or personalized help for writing personal statements through a writing center. While lacking specific experience with editing PA school essays, you may get a nicely polished finished product.

If none of those are options, or you desire professional help, paid editing services are available, such as what we offer through The PA Platform. All editing is done efficiently online and you can be guaranteed that a physician assistant is editing your essay, not an English major or a PA's friend. Most of us have admissions experience as well. We edit for content, grammar, and flow to ensure your essay is ready for submission. Use the code FUTUREPA for a discount on any editing services.

There are a few things to avoid when looking for an editor as well. Do not use any "service" that offers to write your essay or provides a template for you to fill out. This will not be high quality and is also unethical (if you don't write your own essay). Undeniably, there are companies that offer to write your entire essay, and these are ALWAYS a bad idea. No matter what is promised, there is not a specific formula for this essay.

Avoid sending your essay to people you don't know. In The Pre-PA Club Facebook group, on Reddit and various other online resources, I often see people asking for editing help or offering help. There are two main issues to consider: first, you don't know who you're sending your essay to and probability is high they are pre-PA just like you. Secondly, avoid any chance of plagiarism. I've actually heard of this happening in recent years, where your hard work ends up in the hands of someone who will plagiarize it. We like to think the best of people, but the internet allows for anonymity, so keep your guard up. Schools will definitely notice if they receive the same essay from multiple applicants. Also, consider who you're getting advice from. If it's someone in the same situation as you going through the exact same process, they are unlikely to have reliable feedback to share beyond their own personal opinions.

With any feedback you receive, keep in mind that ultimately it is YOUR essay. You have the final say. If you're receiving conflicting advice, take some cooks out of the kitchen and look at the quality of who is giving the advice. Reliance on a few trusted sources should be sufficient for completing a thoroughly edited essay.

Here are some final words on editing; eventually, you have to submit. You could tweak your essay from now on, and never be 100% happy with it. Provided there are no glaring mistakes or issues and you've received positive feedback, go for it! Once you have submitted, don't look back or dwell on your completed essay. Be confident your hard work will pay off.

CHAPTER 7

CHECKLIST

You're so close! This checklist is a great way to verify you're on the right track. Review it before you begin writing and again before you submit. While editing, share this checklist with your editors as well. Considering you've read your personal statement and criticized it a bazillion times, nevertheless it's easy to miss things. Utilize this list to center your thoughts, boost your confidence, and know you're close to submission.

If during this process, you discover parts of the checklist you are unable to confidently check off, no worries. This is a process! Go back, make the necessary changes, and revisit the list. Continue to do this as many times as needed until you feel comfortable with the final product. That being said, at some point, move forward. Call it done and submit. Feeling trepidation after submitting is normal because you'll never feel completely ready. By following the guidelines and checklist, my goal is to provide you with enough guidance to get as close as possible to a perfect essay.

CONTENT

- Does your essay answer the prompt?
- Does everything in your essay relate back to "why PA?"
- Did you adequately explain how you found your interest in medicine/healthcare?
- Did you discuss how you discovered the PA profession?
- Are there clear reasons why you are choosing the PA profession?
- Do discussions of experiences support you as a prepared applicant?
- Do you demonstrate full understanding of the PA profession?
- Do your reasons for being a PA go beyond the "perks' of the profession?
- Did you remove general or generic sentences?
- Does your essay raise more questions than answers?
- Could your essay be applied to any other healthcare profession?
- Did you provide confidence in your ability to complete PA school based on academic success?
- If red flags are presented, are they addressed with a positive outcome?
- Do you have a distinct introduction?
- Do you have a distinct conclusion?
- Is PA mentioned in the first 1/3 of your essay?
- By the end of the essay, does the reader feel like they know you?
- Did you avoid mentioning any specific programs?
- Reapplicants - Were changes made to your original statement?

FORMATTING/EDITING

- Is your essay under 5000 characters including spaces?
- Did you read your essay out loud, record yourself, and listen to the playback?
- Did you remove all tabs?
- Did you avoid special characters or formatting (italics, bold, etc.)?
- Is there a double enter between paragraphs?
- Did you check for repetition (words, phrases, content)?
- Did you write out physician assistant the first time and then use PA throughout?
- If you capitalized Physician Assistant, is it consistent throughout your essay?
- Did you use the correct iterations of PA/PA's/PAs?
- Are abbreviations included that aren't spelled out initially?
- Did you run spell check?

TIME TO SUBMIT

- Do you feel confident in your essay?
- Are you ready for PA school?
- Are you ready to be a PA?
- Have you saved a final copy as a Word document?
- Have you saved a copy elsewhere (Google Drive, email, flash drive, etc.)?
- Are you aware your essay cannot be edited after you submit your CASPA application?
- Are you aware your essay will not carry over between cycles?

PART 4

ESSAY EXAMPLES

CHAPTER 8

ABOUT THIS SECTION

Now you're aware of what to cover in your essay and you have a strong draft, let's look at a few actual essays. The examples chosen for this book show a variety of applicants with different backgrounds, strengths, and weaknesses. In the essay samples, you will see some aspects relating to your experience, however it's unlikely you'll find every essay relevant to your situation. For confidentiality reasons, any personal or identifying information was altered.

It should go without saying; please do not copy or plagiarize these examples. These are not your exact stories, therefore continue to use original words and thoughts throughout this process. Make the essay your own!

In Chapter 9, we'll begin with our first example by showing a before version, one with editing comments, and finally, a completely edited essay. In the subsequent examples, you'll find the original essay, followed by a version with comments. I encourage you to read through the initial essay critically. Make notes and comments about what is done well and any mistakes you pick up on. Thinking through what makes these examples effective will help you evaluate your own essay more objectively.

CHAPTER 9

BEFORE AND AFTER

This first essay comes from a traditional, first-time applicant applying as a junior in college. This applicant has extracurriculars including college athletics, working on campus, and Greek life involvement. Here are their statistics at time of application:

- Overall GPA - 3.6
- Science GPA - 3.4
- Patient care hours - 600
- Healthcare Experience - 300
- Shadowing - 40 hours

This first version is 5,108 characters, so just a little over the limit. For this example, you'll first read the completely unedited version as it was submitted for editing followed by the same essay with comments and editing suggestions. (I promise I didn't change anything prior to editing except for identifying info.) Finally, you'll find a more polished version of this original essay.

BEFORE:

It was a blistering hot July day, seemingly perfect for a refreshing swim in the lake. Joe, at the young age of 81, decided to swim out to the docks to cool off. Once he reached the docks, Joe decided to keep swimming. After treading water for a bit Joe decided to swim back to shore, though he shortly discovered this task was not going to come easily. Since he did not have the endurance that he used to, Joe became very tired and began to struggle, still 50 yards out from shore. Then, he gradually started slipping under the water. His arms and legs burned, his vision was blurry from water entering his eyes, and his chest was tight from lack of air. Right as Joe was about to fully submerge, he felt an arm slip around him and hoist him to the surface and heard a voice asking if he was okay. Joe was relieved, and so was I.

At age fifteen, this was the first time that I saved someone's life. Although my training as a lifeguard prepared me to rescue a drowning victim, I realized I was not prepared to help Joe if he had suffered a heart attack or stroke. As the ambulance had pulled away from the lake, numerous questions swirled in my mind. What diagnoses would be made? What procedures would be performed? If he had a heart attack or stroke, what caused it to happen and how did it affect his body? Could it have been prevented? What would Joe's recovery be? For the remainder of that week, I continued to reflect on Joe and I realized that I had a passion for medicine. I soon began exploring different careers in the healthcare field and the training that would be required to become a physician assistant. I was immediately drawn in by the work/life balance, ability to change specialties, and variety of knowledge that PA's had and kept this in the back of my mind as I entered high school.

Upon starting my undergraduate career, I was certain that I would pursue training as a physician assistant. Therefore, I was focused on engaging in courses that would prepare me for this task. My education at Purple College provided me the opportunity to study subjects such as anatomy and physiology, genetics, kinesiology, nutrition, public health, and exercise physiology. As a small liberal arts school, Purple also challenged me to think holistically by offering a two-semester course called the "Common Intellectual Experience". Throughout the academic year, we diverged in conversations about historical texts, cultures and beliefs, and examined the core questions of the course: what should matter to me, how should we live together, how can we understand the world, and what will I do? The culmination of these courses challenged me to continue to work hard when I failed, to examine things in a new way when I did not understand, and to be resilient. The coursework also challenged me to learn and understand the human body in a scientific manner, but also appreciate that an individual is more than a just a vessel of anatomical structure and function. My passion for science and desire to help and care for others was present when I entered Purple, but my understanding of how beliefs, cultures, and relationships play into medicine was fostered there.

While volunteering at a non-profit organization that treat patients with no insurance, my desire to become a physician assistant flourished. On my first day I was shocked when a patient entered the exam room and explained that they had HIV. The patient was left untreated for the past ten years and now likely had AIDS, Hepatitis C, and possibly tuberculosis. The doctor and physician assistant moved quickly, functioning as a team to order tests, identify necessary medications, and develop an effective treatment plan. When the patient returned to the clinic every 2 weeks, the physician assistant did everything possible to treat this man's medical conditions while getting to know and understand him as a person. By the end of the summer, I had watched the physician assistant successfully treat hundreds of patients using knowledge from many disciplines and developing trusting relationships with both patients and staff, while functioning as a cohesive team with other physician assistants and doctors to deliver the best care possible.

All of my experiences as a student, athlete, and employee drive my ambition to become a physician assistant. My studies have made me versatile, much like a physician assistant, who has the ability to shift their skills and knowledge between different specialties while comprehensively treating all patients they encounter. As a collegiate swimmer, I learned how imperative hard-work, dedication, and team-work are in enabling a successful team effort, which is necessary to deliver quality patient care. As an intern, lifeguard, and tutor I have learned empathy and communication skills and have seen the impor-tance of these attributes in developing trusting patient relationships. I believe becoming a physician assistant will allow me to utilize my knowledge, skills, and abilities to deliver quality patient care as a team member while developing trusting relationships with my patients.

WITH COMMENTS:

It was a blistering hot July day, seemingly perfect for a refreshing swim in the lake. Joe, at the young age of 81, decided to swim out to the docks to cool off. *[This first sentence starts out with good descriptors and a bit of humor with the "young age" comment that actually works, but what's included in the rest of the essay will determine if this informa-tion is relevant enough to stay. At this point, I am inter-ested in the writer's involvement in this situation and their relationship to Joe.]* Once he reached the docks, Joe decided to keep swimming. After treading water for a bit Joe decided to swim back to shore, though he shortly discovered this task was not going to come easily. Since he did not have the endurance **that** he used to, Joe became **very** tired and began to struggle, still 50 yards **out** from shore. Then, he gradually started slipping under the water. His arms and legs burned, his vision was blurry from water entering his eyes, and his chest was tight from lack of air. Right as Joe was about to fully submerge, he felt an arm slip around him and hoist him to the surface and heard a voice asking if he was okay. Joe was relieved, and so was I. *[While dynamic, this story is a bit drawn out, and I still don't really know the writer's role/relationship with Joe. Once we learn that in the next paragraph, it seems a little strange for these descriptions about how Joe was feeling to be from his perspective. This can be shortened greatly with more focus on the applicant. Notice that there are unnecessary words used as well. Taking them out won't change the meaning, but will save on characters. See the after for how this is simplified.]*

At ~~age~~ fifteen, this was the first time ~~that~~ I saved someone's life. *[This wording is strange because it makes me think you have saved other lives, but that is fairly rare. The context with age is helpful though.]* Although my training as a lifeguard prepared me to rescue a drowning victim, I realized I was not prepared to help Joe if he had suffered a heart attack or stroke. As the ambulance ~~had~~ pulled away from the lake, numerous questions swirled in my mind. What diagnoses would be made? What procedures would be performed? If he had a heart attack or stroke, what caused it to happen and how did it affect his body? Could it have been prevented? What would Joe's recovery be? *[I understand what the writer is doing in walking us through how they found an interest in medicine, which is great. This information can be combined with the intro and there's a bit of repetition here.]* For the remainder of that week, I continued to reflect on Joe and I realized ~~that~~ I had a passion for medicine. I ~~soon~~ began exploring ~~different~~ careers in the healthcare field and the training ~~that would be~~ required to become a physician assistant (**PA**). I was immediately drawn in by the work/life balance, ability to change specialties, and variety of knowledge **that** PA's *[should be PAs]* had and kept this in the back of my mind as I entered high school. *[Overall, the info provided is good, but needs some clarification. How did this person find out about PAs and start exploring more? Was it a Google search? This portion is also very wordy and needs pared down. You may also notice a pretty generic list of perks of the PA profession without connection to how it made the writer feel or why they pursued it based on those things. I don't recommend using "work/life balance" as the first reason you are interested in becoming a PA. The abbreviation for PA was not included and then used incorrectly later in the paragraph.]*

Upon starting my undergraduate career, I was certain **that** I would pursue training as a **PA** ~~physician assistant~~. Therefore, I **was** focused on engaging in courses that would prepare me for this task. My education at Purple College provided me the opportunity to study subjects such as anatomy and physiology, genetics, kinesiology, nutrition, public health, and exercise physiology. *[This is an unnecessary list.]* As a small liberal arts school, Purple ~~also~~ challenged me to think holistically by offering a two-semester course called the "Common Intellectual Experience". Throughout the academic year, we diverged in conversations about historical texts, cultures and beliefs, and examined the core questions of the course: what should matter to me, how should we live together, how can we understand the world, and what will I do? The culmination of these courses challenged me to continue to work hard when I failed, to examine things in a new way when I did not understand, and to be resilient. The coursework also challenged me to learn and understand the human body in a scientific manner, but also appreciate that an individual is more than a just a vessel of anatomical structure and function. My passion for science and desire to help and care for others was present when I entered Purple, but my understanding of how beliefs, cultures, and relationships play into medicine was fostered there. *[I'm not seeing how this one specific course has any direct connection to the applicant becoming a PA. This kind of lost me. Occasionally, supplementals will ask for discussion of specific courses, but this space would be used much better if the applicant was emphasizing their academic strengths.]*

While volunteering at a non-profit organization that treat**s** patients with no insurance, my desire to become a **physician assistant** PA flourished. On my first day**,** I was shocked when a patient entered the exam room and explained **that** they had HIV. The patient was left untreated for the past ten years and now likely had AIDS, Hepatitis C, and possibly tuberculosis. *[Discussing volunteering and using examples are both great. This is a situation of being too specific because the conditions mentioned aren't necessarily related to having HIV. It is unclear what this person's role was in the clinic.]* The doctor and **physician assistant PA** moved quickly, functioning as a team to order tests, identify necessary medications, and develop an effective treatment plan. When the patient returned to the clinic every 2 weeks, the **physician assistant PA** did everything possible to treat this man's medical conditions while getting to know and understand him as a person. By the end of the summer, I had watched the **physician assistant PA** successfully treat hundreds of patients using knowledge from many disciplines and developing trusting relationships with both patients and staff, while functioning as a cohesive team with other **physician assistants PAs** and doctors to deliver the best care possible. *[This is good! There's a specific example (even if it needs a little polishing) and I'm seeing how this applicant has interacted with PAs to understand their function. I need to see more of how what the writer saw connects with what they want out of a profession as a PA.]*

~~All of~~ my experiences as a student, athlete, and employee drive my ambition to become a physician assistant. My studies have made me versatile, much like a physician assistant, who has the ability to shift their skills and knowledge between different specialties while comprehensively treating all patients they encounter. As a collegiate athlete, I learned how imperative hard-work, dedication, and team-work are in enabling a successful team effort, which is necessary to deliver quality patient care. As an intern, lifeguard, and tutor I have learned empathy and communication skills and have seen the importance of these attributes in developing trusting patient relationships. I believe becoming a physician assistant will allow me to utilize my knowledge, skills, and abilities to deliver quality patient care as a team member while developing trusting relationships with my patients. *[I stopped changing "physician assistant" to PA because you get the point, but that will save on a lot of characters. Overall, this is a pretty good conclusion. I would like a more clear statement of academic success. Most of our main questions have at least been touched on, but need more clarification. I'm not sure what the actual role was in a PCE/HCE setting, and I can't quite confidently say that this person is fully prepared and passionate about becoming a PA specifically because there isn't enough personal information.]*

AFTER:

In this edited version, notice how the wording is simplified, but doesn't change the overall meaning. The focus is shifted to the writer with more detail to provide a complete picture. This comes in at 4,510 characters.

It was a blistering July day, seemingly perfect for a refreshing swim in the lake. Joe, at the young age of 81, decided to swim out to the docks. While holding my post as a lifeguard, I noticed Joe slipping under the water. I instantly jumped into the water and reached him in time to hoist him to the surface. At age fifteen, I didn't expect to save someone's life. Although my training prepared me to rescue a drowning victim, I realized I was not prepared to help with true medical issues. As the ambulance pulled away from the lake, numerous questions swirled in my mind. What diagnoses would be made? What procedures would be performed? If he had a heart attack or stroke, what caused it and how did it affect his body? Could it have been prevented? Through that week, my reflections led me to realize a passion for medicine. I began exploring careers in the healthcare field and the training required. Through my internet searches, I found the physician assistant (PA) profession, and I was immediately drawn in. The variety of knowledge that PAs gain during their education and flexibility of career options as a PA stayed in the back of my mind throughout high school.

Upon starting my undergraduate career, I continued to pursue steps towards becoming a PA by starting my Biology degree. While my coursework challenged me, I learned to understand the human body in a scientific manner. The culmination of these courses taught me to continue to work hard when I failed, to examine things in a new way when I did not understand, and to be resilient. As a college athlete, I learned to manage my time to prioritize my studies and adjust my study methods when needed. While my academic success has prepared me for PA school, my passion for science and desire to help and care for others was present when I entered Purple, but my understanding of how beliefs, cultures, and relationships play into medicine was fostered there. To confirm my desire to work in medicine, I started volunteering and working as a certified nursing assistant (CNA), which also allowed for direct observation of PAs in action.

While volunteering at a non-profit clinic for non-insured patients, my desire to become a PA flourished. On my first day of working with the PA, Haley, I encountered a patient with a history of untreated HIV over many years. After I gathered vitals and took a history, Haley moved quickly to order tests, identify necessary medications, and develop an effective treatment plan, and consulted with the doctor on her team for reassurance. Through my time at the clinic, I learned how to effectively communicate with patients and elicit the information needed for a more productive visit. I also saw the needs of my community when it comes to a lack of access to healthcare. As a PA, I hope to fill in those gaps to provide comprehensive care to patients who may not know where to seek help.

When our patient returned every 2 weeks, Haley did everything possible to treat this man's medical conditions while getting to know and understand him as a person. By the end of the summer, I watched her successfully treat hundreds of patients using knowledge from many disciplines and developing trusting relationships with both patients and staff, while functioning as a cohesive team with other PAs and doctors to deliver the best care possible. My passion for following my high school dream of becoming a PA became more real as I started to picture myself in the role of a PA. I've always enjoyed working with groups as a team player, but I feel limited by the amount of knowledge and scope of my current position as a CNA. I feel ready for the rigorous nature of PA school, and excited for the education necessary to make an impact on the patients I want to help more thoroughly.

All of my experiences as a student, athlete, and employee drive my ambition to become a PA. My studies have made me versatile, much like a PA, who has the ability to shift their skills and knowledge between different specialties while comprehensively treating all patients they encounter. As a collegiate athlete, I learned how imperative hard-work, dedication, and teamwork are for a successful team effort, which is necessary to deliver quality patient care. As an intern, lifeguard, and tutor I have learned empathy and communication skills. Becoming a PA will allow me to utilize my knowledge, skills, and abilities to deliver quality patient care as a team member while developing trusting relationships with my patients.

CHAPTER 10

STILL IN UNDERGRAD

This next example comes from a student who is currently in undergrad, but applying to PA school as a junior with hopes of skipping a gap year. It's easy to fall into a trap of comparing your lack of experience to other applicants, but emphasizing strengths will be key in showing you're ready to take on PA school. This essay is 5,158 characters.

- Overall GPA - 3.7
- Science GPA - 3.7
- Patient care experience hours - 800
- Healthcare experience - 350
- Volunteer hours - 200
- GRE - 316

ORIGINAL:

I was standing directly across the surgeon, my eyes glued on his steady and precise hands, slowly making incisions along the patient's hair line, ear, and chin. This was the first time I ever saw a surgery and I was about to get a glimpse of the inside of a human face. That day, I was shadowing a plastic surgeon and his PA and watched them perform a rhytidectomy, more commonly known as a facelift. Before entering the operating room, the surgical PA warned that the procedure is quite invasive and to let her know if I did not feel well at any moment. My eyes were fixed to the table for hours with amazement. In this moment, I realized how much I truly love medicine. Viewing these exposed anatomical structures felt surreal and left me breathless.

During this shadowing experience, I spent most of my time with the PA which led to my interest in the career. She had her own cohort of patients and worked with the supervising physician as a team during surgery. She was skillful both in the operating room, as well as at the bedside, addressing all the patient's needs and make sure the clinic operated smoothly and efficiently. As I learned more about her background, she explained that she had worked as an OBGYN PA and an emergency room PA prior to pursuing plastic surgery. I was immediately intrigued. She was able to help such a broad range of people with a broad range of issues while also getting to explore medicine in so many different ways. This flexibility to take on new challenges and explore new areas of patient-centered medicine, is a main motivation for pursuing a career as a PA.

The summer after my freshman year of college, I participated in a research and shadowing program in a neonatal intensive care unit to continue my exploration of the healthcare field. Through this shadowing experience, I saw what team-based medicine truly means. There were so many people involved in caring for the infants including physicians, PAs, nurses, social workers, respiratory therapists, lactation consultants, and more. Once again, the unique role of the PA in delivering inpatient medical treatment was inspiring. Having PAs as a member of the healthcare team allowed for better access to care for each infant. The collaborative relationship between the physician and the PAs helped to improve efficiency and quality of care provided to each patient by increasing the amount time and thought that went toward each individual case. I appreciated the PAs level of decision-making ability that encourages critical-thinking but also teamwork and guidance with other healthcare providers. After viewing the role of a PA in a hospital setting, I was even more excited about pursuing the career path. Through my experiences, it became increasingly evident the value that the PA profession has in delivering quality healthcare, and I longed to be part of this movement.

After this shadowing experience, I was committed to pursuing a career as a physician assistant. Since then, I have pursued multiple clinical opportunities including working as a physical therapy aide. As a PT aide, I loved being able to form relationships with patients of all ages and get to know them over time. In the clinic, I also appreciated the patient-centered model of treatment, aimed to help patients achieve their goals such as returning to a competitive sport. Gaining experience in a position where conversation with patients about their goals is a main focus each day has helped me to refine my communication skills and learn ways to demonstrate compassion as a provider. Finally, as a kinesiology student, I was able to apply a lot of my coursework to each patient situation, gaining further understanding of human anatomy and body mechanics through hands on learning. This ability to apply concepts learned in the classroom to clinical situations is an important skill to have as a PA student with the combination of didactic and clinical studies. Although I did enjoy my experience working with patients as a PT aide, I became disinterested in focusing solely on a patient's movement disorder. I desired the challenging role of caring for the entire person. I realized that medical needs change over time, as well as my own interests. My training as a PA will not limit my ability to explore different avenues of medicine.

The day after I watched the rhytidectomy, the same patient was seen in the clinic. She had driven herself there the day after undergoing such a shocking transformation. I was in awe once again. The physician and the PA talked with the patient about next steps, keeping her calm and confident that the surgery was successful. After this experience, I asked the PA about why she chose plastic surgery. She explained that she entered medicine to help people and plastic surgery can bring confidence and happiness to those that may be struggling. Through extensive shadowing experiences, I have come to greatly appreciate the skill and value of the PA profession. My actions have been intentional in my pursuit to become a compassionate yet efficient medical provider, and I look forward to using my skills to better the health of the community.

WITH COMMENTS:

I was standing directly across **[from]** the surgeon, my eyes glued on his steady and precise hands, slowly making incisions along the patient's hair line, ear, and chin. This was the first time I ~~*ever*~~ saw a surgery and I was about to ~~*get a*~~ glimpse **of** the inside of a human face. ~~*That day,*~~ I was shadowing a plastic surgeon and his **physician assistant** *(*PA*)* and watched them perform a rhytidectomy, **more** commonly known as a facelift. ~~*Before entering the operating room, the surgical PA warned that the procedure is quite invasive and to let her know if I did not feel well at any moment.*~~ **My initial concern about handling the gore quickly faded as** my eyes were fixed to the table for hours with amazement. In this moment, I realized how much I truly love medicine. Viewing these exposed anatomical structures felt surreal and **confirmed my desire to become a PA** ~~**left me breathless**~~. **[Overall, this** *is not a bad intro. It's descriptive and introduces PA from the very beginning. There will need to be some backtracking to answer some of the questions to how the writer got to this point. It's clear why they love medicine, and now I need to see why PA and what led them to medicine.]*

During this shadowing experience, I spent most of my time with the PA which led to my interest in the career. She had her own cohort of patients and worked with the supervising physician as a team during surgery. She was skillful both in the operating room, as well as at the bedside, addressing all the patient's needs and ~~make~~ **making** sure the clinic operated smoothly and efficiently. As I learned more about her background, she explained ~~that she had~~ **how she** worked as an OBGYN *[I would say obstetrics or gynecology here instead]* PA and an emergency room PA prior to pursuing plastic surgery. I was immediately intrigued. She ~~was able to~~ help**s** such a broad range of people with a broad range of issues while ~~also getting to explore~~ **exploring** medicine in so many ~~different~~ ways. This flexibility to take on new challenges and explore new areas of patient-centered medicine, is a main motivation for pursuing a career as a PA. *[This paragraph does show me that the writer has a good understanding of the PA profession. There are parts that are a bit wordy and the verb tense is off in a few places. I still have some questions about how this person actually found the PA profession, but they are making personal connections to why they are drawn to the profession. I want to see how this person has taken steps to prepare beyond this decision now.]*

The summer after my freshman year ~~of college~~, I participated in a research and shadowing program in a neonatal intensive care unit to continue my exploration of the healthcare field. Through this shadowing experience, I saw what team-based medicine truly means.

There were so many people involved in caring for the infants including physicians, PAs, nurses, social workers, respiratory therapists, lactation consultants, and more. Once again, the unique role of the PA in delivering inpatient medical treatment was inspiring. Having PAs ~~as a member of the healthcare team~~ allowed for better access to care for each infant. The collaborative relationship between the physician and the PAs ~~helped to~~ improve*d* efficiency and quality of care provided to each patient by increasing the amount *of* time ~~and thought that went~~ toward each individual case. I appreciated the PA's level of decision-making ability that encourages critical-thinking but also teamwork and guidance with other healthcare providers. After viewing the role of a PA in a hospital setting, I was even more excited about pursuing the career path. Through my experiences, it became increasingly evident the value that the PA profession has in delivering quality healthcare~~, and I longed to be part of this movement~~. *[This further expands on understanding the PA profession, but I already knew the writer had direct exposure to PAs. I want to see more focus on how they are prepared now. This gives a little insight into some of their experience, but not quite enough for me to say they are fully ready. And about that last part about being "part of this movement." I understand it can be difficult to avoid redundant wording, but PA is a career/profession/job/role, not really a movement so that reads a little weird.*

After this shadowing experience, I was committed to pursuing a career as a **PA** ~~physician assistant~~. *[This raises a question about the decision making process because I thought they were already committed before this point. Try to avoid getting yourself into a catch-22 like this because it's confusing to the reader.]* Since then, I have pursued multiple clinical opportunities including working as a physical therapy **(PT)** aide. As a PT aide, I loved ~~being able to~~ form*ing* relationships with patients of all ages and get***ting*** to know them over time. In the clinic, I also appreciated the patient-centered model of treatment, aimed to help patients achieve their goals, such as returning to a competitive sport. Gaining experience in a position where conversation with patients about their goals is a main focus each day has helped ***me to*** refine my communication skills and learn ways to demonstrate compassion as a provider. *[This is more of the discussion of experience that I was looking for. I'm learning what they got out of it.]* Finally, as a kinesiology student, I ***applied*** ~~*was able to apply a lot of*~~ my coursework to each patient situation, gaining further understanding of human anatomy and body mechanics through hands on learning. This ability to apply concepts learned in the classroom to clinical situations is an important skill to have as a PA student, with the combination of didactic and clinical studies. Although I ~~***did***~~ enjoy***ed*** my experience working with patients as a PT aide, I became disinterested in focusing solely on a patient's movement disorder. I ~~***desired***~~ ***desire*** the challenging role of caring for the entire person. I realized ***that*** medical needs change over time, as well as my own interests. My training as a PA will not limit my ability to explore different avenues of medicine. *[This last part does a good job of telling me why the writer feels limited in their current position, and how being a PA will resolve that issue. The emphasis on strengths is good in this section, and these are many qualities that make a good PA student or PA.]*

The day after I watched the rhytidectomy, the same patient was seen in the clinic. ~~***She had driven herself there the day after undergoing such a shocking transformation. I was in awe once again***~~. *[This doesn't feel particularly relevant, and since we're trying to cut down on characters, I would just take it out and get to the point. This is also the concluding paragraph so the focus should be on the applicant.]* The physician and the PA talked with the patient about next steps, ~~keeping her calm and confident~~ *while reassuring her* that the surgery was successful. After this experience, I asked the PA about why she chose plastic surgery. She explained that she entered medicine to help people and plastic surgery can bring ~~confidence and~~ happiness to those ~~that may be~~ struggling. Through extensive shadowing experiences, I have come to greatly appreciate the skill and value of the PA profession. My actions have been intentional in my pursuit to become a compassionate yet efficient medical provider, and I look forward to using my skills to better the health of the community **as a PA. [I'm going to give this conclusion a B+. The story aspects are good, but I really want the focus here to be on the applicant. One thing that hasn't been discussed yet in this essay is a direct mention of academic success. I know they were a kinesiology major, but I want to know they did well and how that will translate to PA school.]**

CHAPTER 11

WAY TOO LONG

This essay is way too long. It is 6,426 characters coming from a post-grad applicant a few years out from undergrad who worked through college. The science GPA is slightly low, but the overall GPA is fairly average for accepted students. The amount of hours is impressive and should be highlighted in the essay.

You'll notice how stories can be shortened in this example to remove 1,500 characters and get under the 5,000 character limit. The use of multiple descriptors is a common mistake prevalent in this essay.

- Overall GPA - 3.49
- Science GPA - 3.2
- Patient care experience - 3,000 scribing hours, 500 CNA hours

ORIGINAL:

Being an individual to depend on has always been important to me—as a friend, a leader, and in the future, hopefully, as a Physician Assistant (PA). There have been many times when my friends, my family, my classmates and coworkers have depended on me; but it wasn't until crisis struck in the vast wilderness of Wyoming, that I realized people felt most confident turning to me in a potentially life-or-death situation. Halfway through a ten-day canoe trip, we found ourselves watching an emergency plane fly low overhead and land on the lake that contained the other half of our group. The arrival of the plane meant someone had activated an emergency SOS radio, meant only for seriously grave matters. In that moment, as we all silently rocked in our boats understanding the weight of the situation, our group of eight looked towards our leader, Jospeh. Without hesitation, Joseph looked straight at me and said "you're coming with me."

As we hurried down the strenuous path, I prepared myself for the worst, internally reciting my training for broken femurs, cracked skulls, and drowning. Fortunately, we came to the other side and found no one injured or seriously ill. Regardless, I was honored to be called to act in this emergency. It was then that I realized other people recognized in me what I had always seen in myself: my steadiness during a stressful situation, my reliability as a medically-trained individual, and my ability as a competent leader.

As this experience details, I have always taken the chance on myself whenever faced with a challenge. I have engaged in a fair share of life experiences that have led to my flourishing into a reliable and dependable person. As an individual with a natural inclination to help people, I was drawn to the field of healthcare. Fortunately, through educational exposure to the profession of Physician Assistants during high school, I began to envision this path for myself. I realized the possibility of working in a medical field as not only an integral member of a team, but also a provider with autonomy. Consequently, I chose an undergraduate degree in the health sciences. This choice was intentional, knowing that health sciences would further propel me toward my dream profession.

In adjunct to my education, my work experiences have only bolstered my choice of a career as a PA. As a Certified Nursing Assistant (CNA), I have spent countless hours, bedside in a nursing home, providing personal care to our elderly population. Through my position as a CNA, I developed skills and knowledge that brought me humility, appropriate yet compassionate bedside manner, and time-management and prioritization skills in working with a vulnerable population. Although this was a challenging job, I found it easy to empathize and provide for these senior citizens for the most intimate of their needs. It is not coincidental, however, that I found this part of the job easy; it was not the first time I was relied upon to take care of some one that could no longer adequately do it themselves.

The compassion I hold for the vulnerable and misconceived began in childhood. As the oldest child of three girls, I had a first-hand lens into our mother's battle with alcoholism. I realized at a young age that oftentimes society neglects people that need the most help and that a stigma exists around those battling with mental health and addiction issues. Her struggle with alcohol not only affected my young life, but continued on into my years throughout college affecting me academically at times. This was inconceivably hard to cope with growing up, but I believe it has shaped me into the person I am today, making the work I want to do even more special. Although my mother ultimately lost her battle, through this intimate perspective on mental health, addiction, and lack of regular medical care, I recognized a dire need for representing and caring for those that are vulnerable. This has made my most recent role at First Choice Clinic undoubtedly the most rewarding.

First Choice Clinic is a primary care clinic for adults on Medicare, providing care to patients in largely underserved areas. As a scribe for a nurse practitioner, I have been exposed to a wide breadth of patients and conditions, from chronic disease management to acute infections. It is no secret that psychiatric conditions, alcohol and drug abuse, homelessness and poor hygiene have a high co-occurrence in underprivileged communities. Through our behavioral health, pain management, social work, and outreach teams, First Choice has given me the opportunity to see how patient care can be approached from multiple interdisciplinary aspects, serving to address socioeconomic issues as well as physical ailments. Working so closely with a Nurse Practitioner, I have been able to observe how mid-level providers function on a care team in Primary Care. Understanding her collaboration with the referring provider, seeing the thought processes in approaching patient care, and acknowledging when an issue is beyond her depth of knowledge has deepened my clarity on a Physician Assistant's position within the field. At First Choice Clinic, I have gained insight as to how doctor's offices work, how many people are involved in the care of patients, and how myself, as a PA, would function in this facility.

Physician Assistants are thoroughly trained providers, expected to be able to function on their own and make complex clinical decisions, and just as importantly to cooperate with a team and serve in whatever capacity is needed. Although I am not a PA yet, I have been called upon to serve in many capacities as well as been called to lead. Since my introduction to the PA profession, I have been able to connect many of my experiences, both professional and personal, to how they have shaped me as a person and how they will affect me as a future healthcare provider. My life and personality have forged my compassion for people and driven my choice to serve people in healthcare. Through my education and professional experiences, I have been able to see that the profession of Physician Assistant best suits my collaboration-based approach to problems, my comfort with working independently, and is conducive to my interests in several specialties. Although this is the beginning of my formal medical education, I am confident that I have been on the correct path for many years.

WITH COMMENTS:

Being an individual to depend on has always been important to me—as a friend, a leader, and in the future, hopefully, as a Physician Assistant (PA). *[Love that PA is mentioned from the very beginning and the abbreviation is correct. The wording is a little strange and can be polished. This is a good one to try reading out loud. I would edit to - I value being dependable as a friend, leader, and hopefully a future PA.]* ~~There have been many times when my friends, my family, my classmates and coworkers have depended on me; but~~ it wasn't until crisis struck in the vast wilderness of Wyoming that I realized people felt ~~most~~ confident turning to me in a potentially life-or-death situation. *[This has me hooked, but some of the lists of irrelevant details can be taken out, which will save on space. I want to know why this person was in Wyoming and what the situation was now.]* Halfway through a ten-day canoe trip, ~~we found ourselves watching~~ *I watched* an emergency plane ~~fly low overhead and~~ land on the lake ~~that contained the other half of our group. The arrival of the plane meant~~ *meaning* someone ~~had~~ activated an emergency SOS. ~~radio, meant only for seriously grave matters. In that moment, as we all silently rocked in our boats understanding the weight of the situation, our group of eight looked towards our leader, Jospeh. Without hesitation,~~ **Our leader** ~~Joseph looked straight at me and~~ said "you're coming with me." *[This is tough because the writing here is well done. When the essay is complete, some of these details may get to stay, but right now the characters need to be reduced so anything non-essential has to be cut. This story needs to be concise enough to fit into one paragraph instead of having to go into the next one. I would also try to edit this direct dialogue out and instead just make it clear that the writer was called upon in this scenario.]*

As we hurried down the strenuous path, I prepared myself for the worst, internally reciting my training for broken femurs, cracked skulls, and drowning. Fortunately, we came to the other side and found no one injured or seriously ill. *[This is a little lackluster based on descriptions from the beginning, which shows why it's best to avoid dramatics. One issue is that the writer references their "training," but I have no idea what that includes or why they would be qualified in this situation to help more than anyone else.]* Regardless, I was honored to be called to act in this emergency. ~~It was then that~~ I realized other people recognized ~~in me~~ what I had always seen in myself: my steadiness during a stressful situation, my reliability as a medically-trained individual, and my ability as a competent leader. *[This story demonstrates strengths, but can be shortened greatly. I'm also going back to the prompt and thinking about what this has to do with the writer deciding to become a PA. I think they are inferring that this confirmed their interest in working in medicine, but that fact could be stated more clearly.]*

As this experience details, ~~I have always taken the chance on myself whenever faced with a challenge.~~ I have engaged in ~~a fair share of~~ life experiences that have led to my flourishing into a reliable ~~and dependable~~ person. As an individual with a natural inclination to help people, I was drawn to the field of healthcare. *[Interest in medicine. Check! Good example of someone who doesn't necessarily have a light bulb moment. Honestly, we could take the first sentence of the essay, summarize the Wyoming story into 1-2 sentences, and jump straight into this as an intro and the essay would be just as dynamic, if not more.]* Fortunately, through educational exposure to the **PA** profession ~~of Physician Assistants~~ during high school, I began to envision this path for myself. *[How they initially found out about PAs - a little vague, but it's there]* I realized the possibility of working in a medical field as ~~not only~~ an integral member of a team, but also a provider with autonomy. Consequently, I chose an undergraduate degree in ~~the~~ health sciences. ~~This choice was intentional, knowing that health sciences would~~ **to** further propel me toward my dream profession. *[This fills in some of the gaps from the intro and at least touches on the main questions we want to see addressed. One issue here is that what you major in can be somewhat arbitrary since the requirements and coursework varies between undergrad institutions. "Health sciences" is fairly broad, so more personal info about how this person performed in coursework would be more helpful.]*

In adjunct to my education, my work experiences have ~~only~~ **bolstered** *[strange word choice]* my choice of a career as a PA. As a Certified Nursing Assistant (CNA), I have spent countless hours, bedside in a nursing home, providing personal care to our elderly population. *[The hours aren't countless and the number is on your application. Be specific, not dramatic.]* Through my position ~~as a CNA~~, I developed skills ~~and knowledge~~ that brought me humility, ~~appropriate yet~~ compassionate bedside manner, and time-management ~~and prioritization~~ skills in working with a vulnerable population. *[Good example of needing to choose just one descriptor.]* Although this was a challenging job, I found it easy to empathize and provide for ~~these~~ senior citizens for ~~the most~~ intimate ~~of their~~ needs. It is not coincidental, however, that I found this part of the job easy; it was not the first time I was relied upon to take care of some one that could no longer adequately do it themselves. *[Highlighting experience is helpful, and the writer's role has been explained well here. The timeline is a little all over the place and could possibly use some reorganization to come up with a more chronological flow.]*

The compassion I hold for the vulnerable ~~and misconceived~~ began in childhood. *[Now, we seem to be going backwards.]* As the oldest ~~child~~ of three girls, I had a first-hand lens into our mother's battle with alcoholism. I realized at a young age that oftentimes society neglects people that need the most help and ~~that~~ a stigma exists around those battling with mental health and addiction issues. *[This is tough. I appreciate the vulnerability and personal insights. These types of details/stories that come from a very sensitive place will make this essay more memorable and give an inside look into why the writer has certain perspectives or goals.]* Her struggle with alcohol not only affected my young life, but continued ~~on into my years~~ throughout college affecting me academically at times. *[Having a timeline is helpful. This mention of academics makes me think there were times where the writer struggled. I would either want this explained a bit more or followed by a very strong, confident statement about ability to overcome academically as well.]* This was inconceivably hard to cope with growing up, but I believe it has shaped me into the person I am today, making the work I want to do ~~even~~ more special. Although my mother ultimately lost her battle, through this intimate perspective on mental health, addiction, and lack of regular medical care, I recognized a dire need for representing and caring for those that are vulnerable. This has made my most recent role at First Choice Clinic undoubtedly the most rewarding. *[Good transition from how a personal experience has impacted decisions moving forward. Having this background may have played a role in the writer's initial interest in medicine, and I would like to see that clearly mentioned if it is the case.]*

~~First Choice Clinic is a primary care clinic for adults on Medicare, providing care to patients in largely underserved areas.~~ *[This would be great for experience details, but for the personal statement has a bit too much of a "tell" vs "show" feel. Adding those details throughout this section would be more effect and save space.]* As a scribe for a nurse practitioner, I ~~have been exposed to~~ *see* a wide breadth of patients and conditions, from chronic disease management to acute infections. *[Example of verb tense. Since this appears to be a current position, present tense verbiage is preferable.]* It is no secret that psychiatric conditions, alcohol and drug abuse, homelessness and poor hygiene have a high co-occurrence in underprivileged communities. Through our behavioral health, pain management, social work, and outreach teams, First Choice has given me the opportunity to see how patient care can be approached from multiple interdisciplinary aspects, serving to address socioeconomic issues, as well as physical ailments. *[This is a little too general with too many lists. These details would be great on the application in experience details, but for the purpose of this essay, I want to know primarily how the writer has been involved and what they have gained from choosing to work in this setting.* Working ~~so~~ closely with a Nurse Practitioner, I ~~have been able to observe~~ *understand [simplify wording as much as possible]* how mid-level providers function on a care team in Primary Care. *[Hold up. Red flag. Try to avoid "mid-level" as it is seen as outdated language surrounding the PA or NP professions. Stick with Advanced Practice Provider if you're looking for a more general term.]* Understanding her collaboration with the referring provider, seeing the thought processes in approaching patient care, and acknowledging when an issue is beyond her depth of knowledge has deepened my clarity on a Physician Assistant's position within the field. At First Choice Clinic, I have gained insight as to how doctor's offices work, how many people are involved in the care of patients, and how myself, as a PA, would function in this facility. *[This is confusing as the reader. While NPs and PAs are very similar, they are not interchangeable and there are differences. I would avoid making a direct parallel like this and inferring that because you've spent time with an NP, you now understand the PA profession. Shadowing/working with other healthcare professionals is invaluable, but doesn't replace direct contact with a PA during your journey.]*

~~Physician Assistants~~ **PAs** are thoroughly trained providers, expected to ~~be able to~~ function on their own and make complex clinical decisions, and just as importantly ~~to~~ cooperate with a team and serve in whatever capacity is needed. *[Addressing the teamwork aspect is very important.]* ~~Although I am not a PA yet, I have been called upon to serve in many capacities as well as been called to lead.~~ *[This sentence feels too general overall, so I would recommend removal.]* Since my introduction to the PA profession, I have ~~been able to~~ connect**ed** many of my experiences, both professional and personal, to how they ~~have~~ shaped me as a person and how they will affect me as a future healthcare provider. My life and personality have forged my compassion for people and driven my choice to serve people in healthcare. Through my education and professional experiences, I ~~have been able to~~ see that the profession of ~~Physician Assistant~~ **PA** best suits my collaboration-based approach to problems, my comfort with working independently, and is conducive to my interests in several specialties. Although this is the beginning of my formal medical education, I am confident ~~that~~ I have been on the correct path for many years. *[Overall, good conclusion. It emphasizes strengths and is passionate. One thing that is missing from this essay is a direct, positive mention of academic success and ability to handle PA school. I would like to see that mentioned more clearly at some point, especially if the mention of struggles is included.]*

CHAPTER 12

NON-TRADITIONAL APPLICANT

Let's hear from a nontraditional, first-time applicant. This person is 46 years old with concerns about GPA and inconsistent volunteer experience. They are also a single parent and have a lot of information they would like to include in the essay. This essay is 4,958 characters.

With many non-traditional applicants, it's common to have a lower overall or science GPA. Presenting improvement in more recent coursework after a change in motivation is important. For a career change, showing full dedication towards PA is imperative.

- Overall GPA - 3.17
- Science GPA - 3.06
- Last 60 hours GPA - 3.9

ORIGINAL:

"Piper One Four Zero November Delta cleared to land runway three five right." On final approach for the runway, heart pounding, I touched down with only one moderate bump and not the bouncing ball technique of my first few landings as a new student pilot at UF. I had successfully navigated to three other airports on my first solo cross-country. It was thrilling and terrifying all at once. Not known for my keen sense of direction, I was immensely relieved. This was the beginning of my adult life and my long journey to becoming a physician assistant. It's taken many years and many invaluable experiences to get here.

Flying is great fun and great responsibility. I have an innate ability to remain calm under pressure and handle stressful situations. As a surgical tech on the thoracic and vascular team, I am on-call regularly. 3am, Saturday morning my phone rang again. I had already been called in twice since the end of my Friday shift and I was dragging. I rushed to the hospital, changed into my scrubs and headed to the OR. The patient had a AAA and was hemodynamically unstable. Massive blood transfusion protocol was enacted. We transfused around more than 60 units of blood product. Mr G survived, due to every person on that team working together, from the surgeons performing the repair to the resident and PA assisting and me keeping the instruments and supplies coming, to the circulator, the runner, and the lab techs each doing their job. Situations like these require calm purposeful action and critical thinking skills. Every day I think of how lucky I am to be part of such an incredible team making a direct impact on the lives of many. As a PA, I will be able to take an even greater role in diagnosis and treatment and I am so excited about this.

Growing up with parents that barely finished high school, college was neither encouraged nor supported. I was on my own. 53 hours into flight training, financial aid ran out and I found myself delivering pizza in my 73 SuperBeetle with no heat, in North Carolina, in the winter, living paycheck to paycheck. Naturally, I answer an ad in the classifieds and move to San Francisco. I had never been there before, but it had to be better than North Carolina in January. Over the next two years in California, I learned how to make my way around the city like a local, and how to get a free lunch by making friends with the extras on a movie set.

Life goes on. Marriage, baby, divorce. Coming home after a double shift to find my 1-year old daughter awake and crying with her father passed out in his chair, I made the decision to leave, wanting a better childhood for her than what I had. I picked her up, walked out and did not look back. Returning to school as a single parent, things were going well. As an undergrad biological anthropology student, I managed to get permission to enroll in the gross anatomy and embryology course with the med students at the university. This moment marked the time that I began to believe that a career in medicine was something I might be capably of having. Not long after gross anatomy, my degree progress was interrupted by financial hardship and significant health issues. A future in medicine was on hold. Volunteering at my daughter's school led me into a prolific career as a professional photographer. As a photographer, I've been witness to many incredible talents and people following their passion. I was so fortunate to be able to spend a lot of time with my daughter, to be a good role model for her and provide a stable, loving home. There were many dark days financially, but we made it through. I know what it is like to pay for $3 of gas at a time, all in pennies, nickels, and dimes.

It took a while, and I do miss my beetle and the old jeeps that followed but I now have a reliable car, an incredible daughter thriving in college, and job in healthcare that has allowed me to work on a collaborative team with MDs, PAs, RNs, and CRNAs. I have seen the roles that each person has. A career as a PA is exactly what I want, and PA is what I am well suited for. For me, PA is the perfect mix of diagnosis, treatment, and collaboration. I love what I'm doing, working in surgery with a talented and compassionate team of providers. It is a privilege to be able to part in saving someone's life, to help them on their worst day and at their most vulnerable. I have had the honor of holding someone's hand as they underwent awake intubation, helped to bring new life, felt the pain of losing a patient, and the thrill of good news. Being in the OR has been like those days in the cockpit...exciting, a little bit scary but now with purpose. I'm ready to do more; to work alongside of physicians, helping to diagnose, treat, and educate patients. Each experience over the course of my life has contributed to making me well-prepared for a career as a PA. I wouldn't change a thing. I'm grateful for every moment, all the joy, all the pain.

WITH COMMENTS:

"Piper One Four Zero November Delta cleared to land runway three five right." On final approach for the runway, heart pounding, I touched down with only one moderate bump and not the bouncing ball technique of my first few landings as a new student pilot at UF. *[This is interesting! I'm already intrigued to know how the writer went from pilot to PA.]* I ~~had~~ successfully navigated to three other airports on my first solo cross-country. It was thrilling and terrifying all at once. Not known for my keen sense of direction, I was immensely relieved. This was the beginning of my adult life and my long journey to becoming a physician assistant (**PA**). It's taken many years and ~~many~~ invaluable experiences to get here. *[I'm feeling a little bit of confusion here. I'm not sure if flying was a career or maybe a hobby? I definitely can't see yet how it connects to being a PA, or even medicine. It's great that PA is mentioned early, but this intro needs more detail about why this experience is relevant to the PA part of the journey.]*

Flying is great fun and great responsibility. I have an innate ability to remain calm under pressure and handle stressful situations. *[Good strengths, still not following the time-line/connections.]* As a surgical tech on the thoracic and vascular team, I am on-call regularly. *[Great patient care experience. I want to know how the person got there.]* 3am, Saturday morning my phone rang again. ~~I had already been called in twice since the end of my Friday shift and I was dragging.~~ I rushed to the hospital, changed into my scrubs and headed to the OR. The patient had a AAA and was hemodynamically unstable. Massive blood transfusion protocol was enacted. We transfused around more than 60 units of blood product. Mr. G survived, due to every person on that team working together, from the surgeons performing the repair to the resident and PA assisting and me keeping the instruments and supplies coming, to the circulator, the runner, and the lab techs each doing their job. *[There's a bit too much going on here. It's more important for the writer to emphasize their role and relate it to how they function on the team instead of discussing what everyone was doing.]* Situations like these require calm purposeful action and critical thinking skills. Every day, I think of how lucky I am to be part of such an incredible team making a direct impact on the lives of many. As a PA, I will ~~be able to~~ take an even greater role in diagnosis and treatment and I am so excited about this. *[This tells me a little more of what the writer wants to do as a PA, but I could use more detail about how they feel limited in their current role. Is it knowledge or skill related? I have some unanswered questions at this point too. Where did the interest in medicine come from? How did they end up working as a surgical tech? Was it in preparation for becoming a PA or is that where their initial exposure to PAs came from? The writing, descriptions, and storytelling are good so far, but flow and details can use some work.]*

Growing up with parents that barely finished high school, college was neither encouraged nor supported. I was on my own. *[These are good personal details.]* 53 hours into flight training, financial aid ran out and I found myself delivering pizza in my 73 Super-Beetle with no heat, in North Carolina, in the winter, living paycheck to paycheck. *[I would try to simplify/condense the details here.]* Naturally, I answer an ad in the classifieds and move to San Francisco. I had never been there before, but ~~it had to be better than North Carolina in January.~~ Over the next two years in California, I learned how to make my way around the city like a local, and how to get a free lunch by making friends with the extras on a movie set. *[This last comment has a weird vibe to me. I don't see how it's relevant to becoming a PA at all. This whole section, while adding personal background details, doesn't seem to relate back to the prompt. This info could be incorporated elsewhere in the essay.]*

Life goes on. Marriage, baby, divorce. Coming home after a double shift to find my 1-year old daughter awake and crying with her father passed out in his chair, I made the decision to leave, wanting a better childhood for her than what I had. I picked her up, walked out and did not look back. *[This also gives insight, but it's starting to feel a bit dramatized at times. Keeping things factual and straightforward would be ideal in this situation. Note - this writer has volunteered the information that they are a parent, which is likely an important part of their life and worth discussing, but this makes that information fair game for an interview.]* Returning to school as a single parent, things were going well. As an undergrad biological anthropology student, I managed to get permission to enroll in the gross anatomy and embryology course with the med students at the university. This moment marked the time that I began to believe that a career in medicine was something I might be ~~capably~~ **capable** of having. *[I would love to know this information much sooner in the essay!]* Not long after gross anatomy, my degree progress was interrupted by financial hardship and significant health issues. A future in medicine was on hold. Volunteering at my daughter's school led me into a prolific career as a professional photographer. As a photographer, I've been witness to many incredible talents and people following their passion. I was so fortunate to ~~be able to~~ spend a lot of time with my daughter, to be a good role model for her and provide a stable, loving home. There were many dark days financially, but we made it through. ~~I know what it is like to pay for $3 of gas at a time, all in pennies, nickels, and dimes.~~ *[We're learning a little more, but I still want to know more of the details behind how/why these decisions were actually made. Career changes are so common to PA, but use caution in showing too much indecisiveness and make the reasons very clear for why you transitioned into different roles or towards PA. By the end, it should be very clear why the writer is confident that PA will fulfill everything they've been missing in other career choices.]*

It took a while, ~~and I do miss my beetle and the old jeeps that followed~~ but I now have a reliable car, an incredible daughter thriving in college, and job in healthcare that has allowed me to work on a collaborative team ~~with MDs, PAs, RNs, and CRNAs. I have seen the roles that each person has~~. A career as a PA is exactly what I want, and PA is what I am well suited for. For me, PA is the perfect mix of diagnosis, treatment, and collaboration. *[It's been mentioned that the writer worked with PAs, and they state that they know what PAs do, but it hasn't really been demonstrated.]* I love what I'm doing, working in surgery with a talented and compassionate team of providers. It is a privilege ~~to be able to~~ **play a** part in saving someone's life, to help them on their worst day and at their most vulnerable. ~~I have had the honor of holding someone's hand as they underwent awake intubation, helped to bring new life, felt the pain of losing a patient, and the thrill of~~

~~good news.~~ *[This feels a little overkill at this point.]* Being in the OR has been like those days in the cockpit; exciting, a little bit scary but now with purpose. *[This reminds me that I'm still not sure how being a pilot plays into becoming a PA.]* I'm ready to do more; to work alongside ~~of~~ physicians, helping ~~to~~ diagnose, treat, and educate patients. *[Missing the mark here and not making me feel confident that the writer understands how PAs function. This seems like it is indicating that PAs are just "helping," but it's so much more involved. I do appreciate that they are covering how they feel limited currently and trying to show how PA will help.]* Each experience over the course of my life has contributed to making me well-prepared for a career as a PA. ~~I wouldn't change a thing. I'm grateful for every moment, all the joy, all the pain.~~ *[Avoid the sentimental or dramatic at the end, and stick to a strong ending surrounding you becoming a PA. Overall, this essay has passion, but it's a little scattered and I have some unanswered questions. The focus needs to be shifted back to "why PA?" more for me to feel confident in the career change.]*

CHAPTER 13

REAPPLICANT

Reapplying is common, and that's why Chapter 2 was devoted to what to do about your essay if you find yourself in that situation. Here are slightly different examples from the previous ones. This first example is from this applicant's first application cycle. Next, you'll find their revamped version for the second application cycle when they were accepted. These are the polished essays ready for submission. Here are the stats from the second application cycle. The only changes were more hours and continued coursework with good grades.

- Overall GPA - 3.53
- Science GPA - 3.51
- Transcripts - 2 Cs, 1 C+, 1 D+
- GRE - 154 Verbal, 144 Quantitative
- HCE - 2,000 hours as front office assistant
- PCE - 14,000 hours as medical assistant
- Leadership - 300 hours
- Volunteer - 300 hours

FIRST CYCLE:

Sometimes you don't know the path life will take. If you were to ask me from elementary school through high school who I would be when I grew up, the answer was always "The next Katie Couric!" Many friends signed my senior yearbook with "Can't wait to see you on The Today Show!" and all I wanted was to be on television. Through the years, my love for interacting with people and telling stories has changed since those days of wanting to be a news anchor. During college, I was unsure of what career I wanted in the field of communication, and majored in Public Relations. With a strong desire to give back and benefit the community around me, after graduation I pursued a career in the realm of nonprofit organizations. Unable to find my desired position, I found myself working for a dermatologist soon after college. I was hired as an office assistant and would be working as a medical assistant with the physician one morning a week. This was my first exposure to working in the medical field, and I enjoyed learning the intricacies of a medical office. Looking back, answering phone calls and managing a physician's schedule gave me valuable knowledge into how a medical office should function. The most enjoyable part of my job were the mornings I worked with the physician. From interacting with patients to learning more about dermatology through observing the physician examine a patient, I began to see myself having a career in the field of medicine.

I do not come from a medical background, but medicine has always interested me. I was diagnosed with Turner's Syndrome and scoliosis when I was going into middle school. My middle school years were marked by traveling to doctor's appointments all over the state, procedures, and medications. As a young teenager, these were some of the most formative years of my life. Being faced with these diagnoses at a young age taught me to have strength during adversity and helped me develop a more positive outlook during hard times. Being placed into the medical field after college was not what I had planned, but taught me more than I ever could have expected.

My first experience with a Physician Assistant (PA) was when the dermatology office hired a PA and I became her medical assistant. Interacting with patients and seeing firsthand how a PA cares for and treats their patients has been my favorite aspect of my job. I have worked with two PAs and can see how the quality of their education impacts how they practice medicine. Following them both straight out of PA school, I was surprised at how much knowledge they brought into our clinic. I have shadowed several other PAs and I'm impressed at the wide range of knowledge they bring into their jobs. Most of the exposure I've had in the medical field has been in dermatology, but shadowing PAs in different specialties has shown me just how valuable a PA can be in any healthcare setting. One of the most enjoyable experiences I had shadowing a PA was in the hospital setting. I saw how a PA managed a fast-paced schedule and variety of patients during the course of a day.

Each day I sit in the passenger seat and watch how a PA can impact and benefit a patient's life through medicine. There are many aspects of being a PA I find attractive, and a main one is the interaction between PAs and their collaborating physician. Through my work experience and shadowing, I appreciate the benefit of a good relationship and the opportunity for continued education and another mind to bounce ideas off of. The experience of working closely with a PA for the past five years has shown me this is something that I want to do for a lifetime. It was overwhelming thinking about going back to school and continuing to work full time, but I do not want to look back and regret not chasing this dream. There are many times I feel limited in my role as a medical assistant, such as the ability to make direct decisions regarding a patient's care, as well as performing advanced procedures.

Sometimes taking the first step is the hardest, and for me and my pursuit of becoming a PA, this was going back to school to complete prerequisite classes. After being out of college for 6 years, I was nervous about going back into the classroom. It was difficult at first, but has taught me lessons in time management and hard work. One of the most enjoyable aspects of going back to school has been the opportunity to continue learning, something I have always enjoyed. I understand how these classes have helped me become a better medical assistant through gathering more knowledge of medical terminology and the anatomy of the human body.

Having the opportunity to become a PA student would be the biggest accomplishment of my life. I have maintained a high GPA while working full time and observed the impact a PA can have on a patient on a daily basis. The opportunity and privilege of serving those who need it most and improving the quality of life of those around me is what I want my life to be characterized by. My degree in Public Relations has allowed me to connect and communicate with patients I interact with every day. The past six years in the healthcare industry and the past five years of being a medical assistant full time has given me valuable insight into the medical field and a knowledge of how a PA practices medicine. There is nothing quite like the look and expression on a patient's face whose persistent rash resolves with a PA's treatment. I want to be a PA in order to improve the quality of people's lives through medicine and I'm ready to begin this journey.

This is a good essay. It's personal, answers all of my questions, and shows passion. There may be a few things that are a bit repetitive, but overall it's ready for submission. When this applicant was not accepted, they had to decide where to make revisions. The next essay is from this applicant's second cycle of applying. Notice the same themes and stories, and how the information is presented differently to make the essay seem new. Pay attention to the inclusion of anything new that changed between application cycles.

SECOND CYCLE:

My introduction to medicine began in middle school when I was diagnosed with Turner syndrome and scoliosis. My sixth grade year was characterized by trips to Children's Healthcare of Arizona every few months. Looking back, I see how these trips during my most formative years shaped me into who I am today. I was a typical 12-year-old girl who loved boy bands and shopping, but also gave myself nightly shots of growth hormone and wore a back brace to school three days a week. Each trip to the hospital started with butterflies in my stomach, but I soon found solace in the nurses and doctors I built relationships with. I was intrigued by the hospital and different departments I was ushered to for tests and appointments. From x-rays in the radiology department and exposure to different special-ties, such as endocrinology and orthopedics, I observed and experi-enced the broad scope of medicine.

As I got older and my trips to CHOA were fewer, I lost touch with those feelings. I viewed healthcare as my personal responsibility, but never as a career I could pursue. Throughout high school and college, I pursued a completely different career path in the field of mass communication. Upon nearing the end of college, I knew this was not what I saw myself doing for the rest of my life. Unsure of what I wanted to do, I found myself working at a dermatology clinic as an office assistant and occasionally as a medical assistant (MA). This was my first exposure to working in the medical field, and I enjoyed learning the logistics of a medical office. Answering phone calls and managing schedules gave me valuable knowledge into how a medical office functions. The most enjoyable part of my job was working with the physician. From interacting directly with patients while taking histories, to learning about dermatology through observing the physician examine a patient, I began to imagine myself with a career in the field of medicine.

After being at my position for one year, the practice decided to hire a physician assistant (PA). My role transitioned into being her

MA full time and I was exposed to this profession in medicine for the first time. I have worked alongside a PA for several years and seen first hand what a PA does day in and day out. The autonomy they have treating patients, the opportunity for lateral mobility, and direct patient care are a few of the aspects of being a PA I find attractive. The interaction between PAs and their supervising physician is something else I look forward to. Through my work experience and shadowing, I have seen the benefit to having a good relationship with your supervising physician and the opportunity for continued education and another mind to bounce ideas off of. I have shadowed PAs that work in hospitals and manage an entire floor of patients, and PAs who work in an Urgent Care where each patient is different than the one before. Even though I work in a specialized healthcare setting, the PAs use their general knowledge of primary care, cardiology, and other fields to best treat their patients, even in dermatology. This is advantageous because when complicated patients are on several different medications, they have the ability to treat them. The experience of working closely with a PA for the past six years has shown me this is something I want to do for a lifetime.

There are many times I feel limited in my role as an MA, such as the ability to make direct decisions regarding a patient's care, as well as performing advanced procedures. The time I spend with a patient discussing treatment plans or taking out sutures are the most enjoyable aspects of being an MA and I am ready and willing for more responsibility when it comes to patient care.

Sometimes taking the first step is the hardest, and for me and my pursuit of becoming a PA, this was going back to school to complete prerequisite classes. This has given me the opportunity to continue learning, something I have always enjoyed. These classes have helped me become a better MA through gathering knowledge of medical terminology and the anatomy of the human body. My degree in Public Relations has allowed me to connect and communicate with the patients I interact with every day. The past seven years I have spent in the healthcare industry and the past six years of being a full time MA has given me valuable insight into the medical field and a knowledge of how a PA practices medicine. I want to use this knowledge I have gained and my unique experiences to treat and manage patients. The opportunity and privilege of serving those who need it most and to improve the quality of life of those around me is what I want my life to be characterized by. The opportunity to become a PA student, and eventually a practicing certified PA, is the best dream I cannot wait to make a reality.

Overall, this version seems more chronological and the descriptions are even better. The storytelling is better. I hope this shows you how the same story can be told differently. The essay now reads as more mature and ready for PA school.

CHAPTER 14

LACKING EXPERIENCE

For full transparency, this is my personal statement. I dug back through the depths of my email inbox to find this beauty, and I actually found a first draft and then my final draft. It's not bad, but there are still mistakes. I clocked in at 4,766 characters for my final draft.

A little background - I applied at the end of my junior year and my biggest issue was low patient care experience hours. I did not expect to get interviews or acceptances that first round. It was 2011 when I applied, and I was a fairly average applicant. These stats haven't changed much since then. I had a ton of volunteer and leadership experience, but I'm unsure of the exact number.

- Overall GPA - 3.58
- Science GPA - 3.48
- GRE - 310
- Patient care hours - 250 as a CNA in a rehab hospital
- Shadowing hours - 150

FIRST DRAFT:

My sister, Anna, who is 3 years younger than me, began having monthly fevers of 104 degrees or more shortly after birth. Many of the medical professionals consulted concluded her condition was mysterious but non life threatening deeming further evaluation was unnecessary. One doctor stands out to me because of the interest he took in my sister's condition. Two years after first seeing Anna and hours of extensive research, Dr.Jones diagnosed her illness as PHAPA, a rare illness with many unknowns, but thankfully not life threatening.

This process assured me that I wanted to work in healthcare and strive to be the type of professional who has a genuine interest in the well-being of my patients. My dad first introduced me to the idea of being a physician assistant during my junior year of high school. The prospect was so intriguing, especially after researching the unlimited opportunities of Physician Assistants. By the time I graduated from high school in 2008 and began my freshman year at UGA, my unwavering goal has been centered on being a PA. For the past four years I have been immersed in rigorous classes, shadowing, CNA training, and in any other means that will help to better prepare myself for a career as a Physician's Assistant.

Freshman year at UGA was extremely difficult: the strenuous science classes, being on my own for the first time, and trying to learn to study efficiently. During this was a period of time I spent a time researching options and asking myself what I really wanted to do for the rest of my life. I got advice from PAs, doctors, family, teachers, and others who knew me well in order to help me discover the best fit for me. Through this process I discovered that my greatest gifts are that I am intelligent, hard working, driven, and totally intrigued with the intricacies of the human body and more importantly, I'm compassionate about helping people. Although independence is important, I enjoy working as part of a team and I believe the idea of an accountability system in healthcare is essential to preventing mistakes thus providing better care to patients. And I'm the type of person who sets goals and will do what it takes to make them happen as soon as possible. to me because I just want to start doing what it is I desire to do.

For the past two years, I have shadowed PAs in the fields of Orthopedics, General Surgery, Dermatology, and Internal Medicine while witnessing many procedures including surgeries. The give and take relationship doctors have with their assistants has been impressive as well as the professionalism exhibited during stressful situations. This was very apparent during one such incident when what was thought to be a small cyst was actually an aneurysm. What could have been a dangerous situation, because of the quick actions of the PA, turned out to be minor. I know with certainty, had I been the PA, I would have handled the situation with the same calm and assurance. Through my CNA license, I have gained further insight into patient care and interaction.

Flexibility, demand, and growth are all attractive aspects of the PA profession, but my interests go beyond these. As a PA, I will utilize my skills, intelligence, and compassion while helping others.

The information presented is good and answers the main content questions, but it's not very dynamic or interesting. This was a very rough first draft, but I did send it to a few family members for input and help with editing and polishing. My final draft is below and with some changes in organization and wording, it's a more engaging, confident essay.

FINAL DRAFT:

If hard work, determination, and focus assure one of success, a career as a physician assistant (PA) is within my reach. Strong work ethic, as well as persistence, have directed my actions. Whether a small thing like learning to ride my bike or making a career choice, I know what I want to accomplish and will passionately strive to obtain this goal.

My aspiration is to be a PA who is compassionate, detail oriented, and conscious of each patient's needs.

My younger sister, Anna, began having monthly fevers exceeding 102 degrees shortly after birth. Many medical professionals who were consulted concluded that her condition was mysterious, but not life threatening. One doctor stands out because of the interest he took in my sister's condition. Two years after he first saw Anna and many hours of extensive research, Dr. Jones diagnosed her illness as PHAPA, a rare disease with many unknowns and no clear treatment.

This exposure to healthcare encouraged me to pursue a career as a professional who holds a genuine interest in a patient's well being. My father introduced me to the PA profession during my junior year of high school. During the next two years, I devoted time towards researching available options in the medical field and asking myself what I really wanted to do for the rest of my life. I sought advice from health professionals, family, and teachers. My greatest strengths are determination, an interest in the intricacies of the human body, and compassion for helping people. As a PA, I will utilize those characteristics in a field that is both challenging and rewarding. After making this decision, I was challenged to step out of my comfort area of literature and social sciences to begin a degree in Biology.

For the past four years at the University of Georgia, I have immersed myself in rigorous classes, observation, certified nursing assistant (CNA) training, and volunteering to prepare myself for a career as a PA. During Spring semester 2011, I drove an hour away every weekend for three months in order to complete the CNA program while I maintained a full time schedule at school.

With my CNA license, I have gained further insight into patient care and interaction. Patients value someone who cares and takes time to explain procedures and complicated medical jargon. Being a CNA before going into a profession as a PA has provided me with valuable insight into the team aspect of medical care. At the rehab hospital, I worked with many nurses, occupational therapists, physical therapists, and doctors to ensure quality care for the patients. Each member has his or her own role, but recovery occurs quickest for the patient when everyone works together to provide the highest quality of care.

To further enhance my understanding of PA responsibilities, I have shadowed in various fields, allowing me to observe interactions between both patient and PA and Physician and PA and procedures, including surgeries. The ranges of independent levels among the PAs and the professionalism exhibited during stressful situations has been impressive. There was one incident when a diagnosis of a small cyst was actually an aneurism in a dermatology office. A dangerous situation was quickly averted because of the quick actions and judgment of the PA.

I have also participated in international volunteer trips with a campus ministry, to Amsterdam and Jamaica. I now see a need for medical care in other countries, and I hope to utilize my knowledge and skills as an international medical provider. For example, the project I worked on in Jamaica was constructing a three-room home to replace the leaking, dirt floored shack occupied by a mother and her five children. She showed her gratefulness with food and tears, while the children showed their excitement with hugs for every-one. This was a small step toward providing this family with a healthier environment. Eventually, I hope to contribute actual healthcare to families such as these.

Flexibility, demand, and growth are all attractive aspects of the PA profession, but my interests go beyond these. As a PA, I will utilize my skills, intelligence, and compassion while helping others. Although self-sufficiency is important, I enjoy working as part of a team, which increases accountability. An accountability system in healthcare is essential to preventing mistakes, thus providing better care to patients. The possibility of working in different areas and specialties as needs change makes this career appealing. I am ready to learn and prepare for my career as a PA.

There are still plenty of things that could use work

here (now that I know better), but it's much more organized and flows better than the first version. The main thing to notice here is how I didn't highlight my lack of patient care hours, but instead focused on the lessons I took out of the experience I had obtained. This statement provides essential information and enough differentiating aspects for a reader to have a good idea of what I completed during undergrad.

CHAPTER 15

GPA ISSUES

This essay comes from a first generation student who is reapplying with a 2.9 GPA. This 28-year-old is continuing to take classes in the evening full-time, while also working full-time. This essay is 4,450 characters.

We have the luxury of knowing grades or GPA were an issue at some point during the writer's education. If I'm reviewing an application and see these kinds of numbers in the GPA sections, I expect to see academics addressed with an explanation in the essay that follows. As you read, determine if there is confidence in how the student has shown improvement in grades despite the GPA calculations.

No other stats were provided outside of the GPA, but we would hope to see a well-rounded applicant in all other areas outside of grades.

ORIGINAL:

"You want to be someone's assistant?" my dad asked, the disappointment palpable. I was raised by immigrant parents who followed all the rules to achieve the unattainable 'American Dream.' In order for this dream to come true for them, my dad left his engineering job became a server at a restaurant, and expected us to all be successful with the stipulation of that success having the title, 'doctor'. May it be a physician, pharmacist, dentist, or even a veterinarian, they weren't too picky as long as it held the prestigious title. For as long as I can remember, becoming a doctor was ingrained in my mind. My responses to the first grade prompts always stated "I want to be a doctor, because I want to help people" with a spelling error or two thrown in.

When I graduated high school, I went to a college not too far, but far enough, and I still did what was expected: biology degree, following a pre-medicine track, and joining Pre-Med Club. As the semesters passed and I was going through the motions, I realized this was never the dream I cultivated for myself. Being just far enough away, I was finally granted some freedom and allowed myself to stray away from the pressure of fulfilling my parents' dreams for me. As any nineteen year old would do, I felt the need to rebel and create my own path.

In the summer of 2013, I volunteered as a medical missionary at the Joy Clinic in Kenya. It was there that I worked with a family medicine Physician Assistant, Haley. I first learned she was a PA when she was called 'doctor', she corrected and educated them with the limited words she knew. She served with such grace and cared so deeply for the patients and the profession. Seeing the local villagers coming to the free clinic with hopes of an answer to an ache or pain or checking to see if their babies were going to live another day was tragic and beautiful at the same time. Although there was a language barrier, I quickly learned the necessary medical words and words of comfort in order to assure the patients they were in good hands.

Volunteering in Kenya did not only consist of taking vitals, administering injections, and performing ultrasounds, there were also days I would visit the children in the orphanage, make meals for those in shelters, support and play with children of incarcerated men, and provide support to widows. Although those were blessings, working in the Joy Clinic was where I grew the most. While working with Haley, we performed an emergency Cesarean section, and she delivered a healthy baby boy to a glowing mother. I learned about her previous experience working in Ob/Gyn, as well as her years working in Emergency Medicine when she first graduated. The way she collaborated with the practicing physician, while still making important calls was inspiring. My experience in Kenya opened my eyes to my new dream and the world of being a PA.

This shift in vision, lead to changing my major and learning as much as I could about becoming a PA. The years following graduation I worked full time and took a full load of night classes to do as much as I could to improve myself. I have shadowed and volunteered on the weekends becoming more engrossed with the life and career path. It lead me to earn an EMT-B certificate, and throw myself into research under brilliant and extremely talented medical providers. I learned a significant amount about pediatric and obstetrics research. I currently work as a Clinical Research Coordinator for the Staircase Center for Alzheimer's Disease & Cognitive Neurology at Treehouse University.

It turns out I did know what I wanted to do in first grade: I want to help people. I want to help in any capacity that is necessary. May the need be in obstetrics or surgery or emergency medicine, I want to be there and fill the need. I don't need the prestige of a certain title, that's something, following in Haley's footsteps, I am willing to correct and show with my demeanor and compassion to each patient. The ability to grow, collaborate, and switch fields would allow me to be a fountain of knowledge and help in more ways than I can dream of. Every experience I have had with a PA, makes it obvious that this is exactly what I am meant to do. They show so much compassion and care for each patient they encounter and it is evident that each patient is in capable hands. Becoming a Physician Assistant is not simply what I want to do, but is something I am meant to do.

WITH COMMENTS:

"You want to be someone's assistant?" my dad asked, the disappointment palpable. I was raised by immigrant parents who followed all the rules to achieve the unattainable 'American Dream.' *[From the start, we get some insight into the background of the writer and possibly their motivations. This does seem a little negative, but may be redeemed as long as there are facts to indicate why the writer has chosen PA despite their parent's wishes.]* In order for this dream to come true for them, my dad left his engineering job, became a server at a restaurant, and expected us to ~~all~~ be successful with the stipulation of ~~that success having~~ the title, 'doctor'. May it be a physician, pharmacist, dentist, or even a veterinarian, they weren't ~~too~~ picky as long as it held the prestigious title. For as long as I can remember, becoming a doctor was ingrained in my mind. My responses to the first grade prompts always stated "I want to be a doctor, because I want to help people" with a spelling error or two thrown in. *[There is passion here from the beginning, but it doesn't seem to be quite the right type. This intro feels a little prickly. There is a lot of focus on family expectations and not as much on what the writer wants to do. Reading further into the essay, I would say ditch this intro, jump into the next section, and add a comment about the parents expectations there.]*

When I graduated high school, I went to a college not too far **away**, ~~but far enough,~~ and I ~~still~~ did what was expected **from my parent's traditional views**: biology degree, following a pre-medicine track, and joining Pre-Med Club. As the semesters passed and I was going through the motions, I realized this was never the dream I cultivated for myself. Being just far enough away, I was ~~finally~~ granted some freedom and allowed myself to stray away from the pressure of fulfilling my parents' dreams for me. As any nineteen year old would do, I felt the need to ~~rebel and~~ create my own path. *[I like this so much better. It's more personal without the negativity attached and helps the story progress. I do want to see where the writer ended up finding their own interest in medicine.]*

In the summer of 2013, I volunteered as a medical missionary at the Joy Clinic in Kenya. *[Great experience. Instead of using "summer of 2013," it would be more helpful to give a description of the timing like "summer after freshman year." The reader may not know how old you are or when you graduated, which makes a random date arbitrary.]* It was there that I worked with a family medicine Physician Assistant (**PA**), Haley. I first learned she was a PA when she was called 'doctor,' she corrected and educated them with the limited words she knew. She served with such grace and cared so deeply for the patients and the profession. Seeing the local villagers coming to the free clinic with hopes of an answer to an ache or pain or checking to see if their babies were going to live another day was tragic and beautiful at the same time. Although there was a language barrier, I quickly learned the necessary medical words and words of comfort in order to assure the patients they were in good hands. *[This paragraph shows how the writer found out about the PA profession very directly and thoughtfully, while incorporating their own impressions and experience.]*

Volunteering in Kenya did not only consist of taking vitals, administering injections, and performing ultrasounds, there were also days I would visit the children in the orphanage, make meals for those in shelters, support and play with children of incarcerated men, and provide support to widows. Although those were blessings, working in the Joy Clinic was where I grew the most. While working with Haley, we performed an emergency Cesarean section, and she delivered a healthy baby boy to a glowing mother. I learned about her previous experience working in Ob/Gyn, as well as her years working in Emergency Medicine when she first graduated. The way she collaborated with the practicing physician, while still making important calls was inspiring. My experience in Kenya opened my eyes to my new dream and the world of being a PA. *[No major changes needed here. The story is progressing, and the writer's passion is becoming apparent. It is a nice shift from the discouraged feel of the current intro. There is also a good demonstration of understanding what the PA profession entails. I need to know the steps taken to move closer to that goal now.]*

This shift in vision, ~~lead~~ **led** to changing my major and learning as much as I could about becoming a PA. The years following graduation I worked full time and took a full load of night classes to ~~do as much as I could to~~ improve myself. I have shadowed and volunteered on the weekends becoming more engrossed with the life and career path. It ~~lead~~ **led** me to earn an EMT-B certificate, and throw myself into research under brilliant and extremely talented medical providers. I learned a significant amount about pediatric and obstetrics research. I currently work as a Clinical Research Coordinator for the Staircase Center for Alzheimer's Disease & Cognitive Neurology at Treehouse University. *[The steps taken are here, but are reading a bit too much just like a list. The rest of the essay is so dynamic, and I would like to see that continue here with more explanation of what the writer's takeaways are from these experiences. How have they prepared them for success?]*

It turns out I did know what I wanted to do in first grade: I want to help people. I want to help in any capacity ~~that is~~ necessary. May the need be in obstetrics or surgery or emergency medicine, I want to be there and fill the need. I don't need the prestige of a certain title, ~~that's something, following in Haley's footsteps,~~ **and** I am willing to correct and show with my demeanor and compassion to each patient. The ability to grow, collaborate, and switch fields would allow me to be a fountain of knowledge and help in more ways than I can dream of. Every experience I have had with a PA, makes it obvious ~~that~~ this is exactly what I am meant to do. They show so much compassion and care for each patient they encounter and it is evident that each patient is in capable hands. Becoming a **PA** ~~Physician Assistant~~ is not simply what I want to do, but is something I am meant to do. *[The passion is back! As a conclusion, the writer's goals are emphasized. The strengths could be included more here. Overall, this essay is on the right track and has most of the info showing understanding the PA profession. We have insider info that the writer's GPA is subpar, and academics have not been addressed at all. It's important to show improvement and mention an upward trend, better grades, or success in the classroom in some fashion.*

I would also like to see a more clear indication of where the writer's interest in medicine came from if it was not a result of their parent's initial pressure. Some clarification is needed to make this a stronger essay.]

CHAPTER 16

PATIENT TO PA

Using personal experiences as a patient isn't a bad technique. This traditional reapplicant has a Biochemistry degree, but these statistics are on the lower side compared to most accepted students. This essay is 4,975 characters.

- Overall GPA - 3.33
- Science GPA - 3.03
- Patient care experience - 170 hours as OB/GYN MA
- Shadowing - 60 hours with a PA, 80 hours international medicine
- Volunteer hours - 75
- Research - 300
- Leadership in multiple organizations

ORIGINAL:

Hip surgery. These two, almost foreign, words bring to mind unfamiliar images of senior citizens in nursing homes for most. Of course, the only people who could ever have hip surgery would be those of at least forty years or older. At least that's what I thought at the young age of only fifteen. Quickly, I realized my naivety as these words became very persistent in my life, facing the OR twice for hip surgeries. The eloquent way healthcare professionals introduced the medical world to me is why I aspire to become a physician assistant.

After enduring two long hip surgeries in high school, my pathway of life changed. This diversion from my previously decided future opened my eyes to a whole new world of possibilities. Through the determination of surgery, I was easily fascinated with the technology used and even more flabbergasted by the advancements made when my doctor and PA began explaining my procedure. Although my arthroscopic surgeries were small in size, they filled my mind with grand amazement as I tried to grasp the fact that a procedure so detailed only left two tiny scars. During these appointments, the care from one particular PA transformed the fear and confusion of a 15-year-old kid into the spark of fascination of my adult aspiration to care for others in need within the healthcare world.

Frustratingly enough, this spark grew as I saw the healthcare world from a patient's point of view, not truly understanding the depths of my case. As a patient, I had so many questions of concern, but had so few healthcare professionals who were able to explain the process in a way I could understand as an inexperienced teenager. Many professionals simply reiterated the medical terminology without fully explaining what each term meant. I struggled until one particular PA was able to see the perplexed look on my face after the doctor left the room. She took it upon herself to sit down with me and explain my procedure in a way to which I was able to relate. Instead of repeating the terms, she broke down each piece of the puzzle to allow me to see the bigger picture clearly. Not only was she able to explain the procedure, she also established a comfortable environment for me to ask questions when I was still confused. This type of patient interaction made me realize how important it is for medical professionals to establish a sense of trust and comfort with patients. This interaction has allowed me to focus on how I can do the same, preventing future patients from experiencing that sense of confused helplessness.

This spark for knowledge began setting fires throughout the entirety of my journey. Once I was rolled into the operating room on the morning of surgery, I felt like a kid in a candy store. I fought the anesthesia in hopes of looking around the OR for just a few more moments to process the experience. Although I failed miserably in staying awake, the questions still gleamed in the back of my mind when I awoke. I began to wonder how each use of technology, medical professional and step of procedure came together, specializing for just one operation. These questions led me to an international shadowing program, allowing me to observe the world of medicine abroad. As I traveled to Greece, the same emotions I first experienced in the OR of my hip surgeries began to magnify as I observed liver transplants, hip replacements, colonoscopies, and even facial reconstructions. Even though I didn't understand the language these medical professionals were speaking during surgery, I fell in love with other means of communication that were required in the OR: the language of medicine.

To understand the language of medicine, I dove into the chemistry and biology of the many wonders of the miraculous thing we call life. At Tabletop University, I found beauty in the combination of chemistry and biology which fueled my fascination with the medical field. I studied many medical research topics, broadening my knowledge and experience in both the chemical laboratory as well as the medical world. My research experience as an undergraduate student allowed me to develop an array of problem-solving skills. Much like the medical world, the research field requires a specific skill set to combat the many unexpected problems that may potentially arise.

As I entered the healthcare world as an OB/GYN medical assistant, I have been able to apply these problem-solving skills to real life scenarios. In combination with my past experience of surgery, volunteering, and shadowing, I have been able to answer some but not all of the questions I pose to myself in relation to the medical world. Although I am certain I don't fully understand everything in regards to life, I aspire to continue my studies as a PA in hopes of keeping my spark for understanding alive. Life is full of both learning and teaching experiences, which I plan to take full advantage of to fuel my desire of helping others in the world of medicine as a PA.

WITH COMMENTS:

Hip surgery. These two, ~~almost foreign,~~ words bring to mind unfamiliar images of senior citizens in nursing homes for most. ~~Of course, the only people who could ever have hip surgery would be those of at least forty years or older~~. At least that's what I thought at the young age of only fifteen. *[I wasn't completely sure who the initial patient the hip surgery was referring to from the beginning. Remember the age range of your likely reader and try to avoid insulting them by referencing them as old.]* Quickly, I realized my naivety as these words became ~~very~~ persistent in my life, facing the OR twice for hip surgeries. The eloquent way healthcare professionals introduced the medical world to me is why I aspire to become a physician assistant **(PA)**. *[PA is mentioned early, and it appears the writer's personal medical experience is what drew them to working in healthcare.]*

After enduring two long hip surgeries in high school, my pathway of life changed. This diversion from my previously decided future opened my eyes to a whole new world of possibilities. *[This feels a little vague since I'm unsure of what their "previously decided future" is referring to. Additional detail on that decision shift would be helpful.]* Through the determination of surgery, I was ~~easily~~ fascinated with the technology used and ~~even more~~ flabbergasted by the advancements made when my doctor and PA began explaining my procedure. *[So far, the wording in this paragraph is a little off/exaggerated. The next part is much more direct.]* Although my arthroscopic surgeries were small in size, they filled my mind with grand amazement as I tried to grasp the fact that a procedure so detailed only left two tiny scars. During these appointments, the care from one particular PA transformed the fear and confusion of a 15-year-old kid into the spark of fascination of my adult aspiration to care for others in need within the healthcare world. *[This also feels like an intro and seems to repeat what was said in the first paragraph. I would choose one or combine the information. I already know the surgery led the writer to want to work in medicine. If this was the writer's first encounter with a PA, I want that to be more clear.]*

Frustratingly enough, this spark grew as I saw the healthcare world from a patient's point of view, not truly understanding the depths of my case. *[The transition of "frustratingly enough" doesn't seem to fit here or flow from the excitement in the previous paragraph.]* As a patient, I had so many questions of concern, but ~~had so~~ few healthcare professionals ~~who~~ were able to explain the process in a way I could understand as an inexperienced teenager. Many professionals simply reiterated the medical terminology without fully explaining what each term meant. I struggled until one particular PA ~~was able to see~~ **noticed** the perplexed look on my face after the doctor left the room. She ~~took it upon herself to sit~~ **sat** down ~~with me and~~ **to** explain my procedure in a way ~~to which I was able to~~ **I could** relate. Instead of repeating the terms, she broke down each piece of the puzzle to allow me to see the bigger picture clearly. Not only was she able to explain the procedure, she also established a comfortable environment for me to ask questions when I was still confused. This type of patient interaction made me realize how important it is for medical professionals to establish a sense of trust and comfort with patients. This interaction has allowed me to focus on how I can do the same, preventing future patients from experiencing that sense of confused helplessness. *[As a PA?? This explanation of the encounter with a PA shows personal interaction and some understanding of the role. It's borderline on being negative about other professions and could be rephrased slightly, but keeps the focus on the relationship between the PA and the patient. I would still like to know more concretely whether this was the first time the writer was introduced to the PA profession.]*

This spark for knowledge began setting fires throughout the entirety of my journey. Once I was rolled into the operating room on the morning of surgery, I felt like a kid in a candy store. I fought the anesthesia in hopes of looking around the OR for just a few more moments to process the experience. *[These analogies are a little strange to me in the setting of going into a surgery.]* Although I failed ~~miserably~~ in staying awake, the questions still gleamed in the back of my mind when I awoke. I began to wonder how each use of technology, medical professional and step of procedure came together, specializing for just one operation. *[We're halfway into the essay and still talking about how the writer found an interest in medicine. That has already been established, so it's time to move on to more PA-specific discussion instead of belaboring this point.]* These questions led me to an international shadowing program, allowing me to observe the world of medicine abroad. As I traveled to Greece, the same emotions I first experienced in the OR of my hip surgeries began to magnify as I observed liver transplants, hip replacements, colonoscopies, and even facial reconstructions. Even though I didn't understand the language these medical professionals were speaking during surgery, I fell in love with other means of communication ~~that were required~~ in the OR: the language of medicine. *[This sounds like an interesting experience, but I'm struggling to see the direct connection to how it relates to the writer becoming a PA. Everything to this point could be simplified to two paragraphs at the most.]*

To understand the language of medicine, I dove into ~~the~~ chemistry and biology ~~of the many wonders of the miraculous thing we call life~~. *[Continuing to get a bit too figurative here, and the next sentence is repetitive after this one. Picking one will suffice.]* At Tabletop University, I found beauty in the combination of chemistry and biology which fueled my fascination with the medical field. I studied many medical research topics, broadening my knowledge and experience in both the chemical laboratory, as well as the medical world. My research experience as an undergraduate student allowed me to develop an array of problem-solving skills. Much like the medical world, the research field requires a specific skill set to combat the many unexpected problems that may potentially arise. *[Coursework and experience is important, but what does it have to do with becoming a PA? We're almost to the end of the essay, but I still have some questions! Beyond one encounter with a PA who communicated well, what else is appealing to the writer about the profession? How does being a PA connect with the writer's aspirations when compared to any other medical career?]*

As I entered the healthcare world as an OB/GYN medical assistant, I have ~~been able to apply~~ **applied** these problem-solving skills to real life scenarios. In combination with my past experience of surgery, volunteering, and shadowing, I have ~~been able to~~ answer**ed** some, but not all, of the questions I pose to myself in relation to the medical world. Although I am certain I don't fully understand everything in regards to life, I aspire to continue my studies as a PA in hopes of keeping my spark for understanding alive. Life is full of both learning and teaching experiences, which I plan to take full advantage of to fuel my desire of helping others in the world of medicine as a PA. *[This is a little fluffy for a conclusion. I would like to see some more facts in regards to preparedness instead of superficial mentions.*

This is a good start, but there are a few core topics missing. I cannot say the writer has a full understanding of the PA profession based on what has been included thus far. I'm also missing any mention of academic strengths and reassurance of a strong scholastic performance that will translate to PA school success.

Using a personal medical scenario can be effective, but should still lead into answering the main content questions.]

CHAPTER 17

PARENT TO PA STUDENT

This is a first time applicant who is also a single parent. She moved to the US when she was young and continued to pursue the PA profession. This essay is 4,879 characters. The GRE score is low, but GPA and hours stated are average for accepted students.

- Overall GPA - 3.45
- Patient care hours - 2,500 as a scribe
- GRE - 284

As a parent, it would feel strange to not mention family, but keep the focus on you as an applicant primarily. Also realize you are volunteering this information to the admissions committee. While they cannot ethically ask about personal information or make a decision based on these facts, the info is fair game if you bring it up.

ORIGINAL:

Growing up in rural Peru greatly impacted my family as my mother struggled to single-handedly raise her three children. Before being blessed with the opportunity to relocate to Dallas, TX at the age of 9, we planned to hike a mountain in Peru with our extended family in anticipation of being separated from them for the next 10 years. Similarly, this hike compared to organizing my first steps for my career. I strictly focused on my core science subjects in my undergraduate years to ensure success for the possibility of graduate school while working full time.

It was a simple march towards my career goals until suddenly, the terrain developed to a steep uphill climb. As I stared down at my positive pregnancy test, I felt the first unsteady footing up this metaphorical mountain in my life. Yet instead of slipping away, I grabbed on to the nearest steady cornerstone and I pulled myself up. Deciding to become a single parent at the age of 19 was ultimately the hardest choice I had to endure but the most profound and proudest moment in my life. I constructed the objective of never allowing my child to be an excuse for my failures. My family roared in applause as I graduated 7 months pregnant with honors for my associates degree at Fruit Snack College. Furthermore, I persevered in my studies at the University of Popcorn the following fall semester after giving birth to my first-born, Melissa, in July of 2015.

Fortunately, I mastered the concept of time management skills and academically excelled in my projects by using balance in my routine. I sustained two jobs as a lifeguard and a medical scribe while completing school as a full-time student and being a single parent. An unexpected, yet amazing outcome of my decision to be a medical scribe was learning about the physician assistant (PA) profession. While working with a PA, I once witnessed the joint effort of a flawless facilitated admission of a woman in labor to the maternity ward. The PA assured all tests including pelvic exams were within normal limits while the physician contacted obgyn department to ensure proper admission. Despite the collaboration between this PA and supervising physician, the course of nature resumed command and conducted the patient dilating from 6 cm to the expulsion of the baby's head in seconds inside the Emergency Department(ED). I was mesmerized by the partnership and trust between these two providers had to succeed in the delivery of a healthy baby. Witnessing the collaboration between the PA and supervising physician solidified my interest in the medical profession and ultimately ignited my interest towards the PA profession.

While scribing for different providers in Central Hospital ED, I was able to work closely with PAs and truly grasp their approach to patient evaluation and care. These PAs would thoroughly investigate past medical history, social history, and previous failed treatments of the patient. Even upon discharge, PAs would extensively educate patients by clarifying ED return symptoms, recommend further evaluation with a specialist, and thoroughly instruct them on prescription use. Additionally, these PAs would insist on prescribing although these medicines could be found over the counter. Each PA would demonstrate compassion, sympathy, and most of all time in guaranteeing patient satisfaction and solicitous education. This established my career towards the PA profession as I also yearned in contributing to overall patient satisfaction through the improvement of bedside manner and assuring the patient emotionally.

After tirelessly researching PA school requirements, I began preparing for my GRE through applying several studying methods to multiply my chances of obtaining my ideal score. Until I experienced a similar downfall to my hike experience in Peru, when I learned of Melissa's half-brother's death. Mentally incapable of continuing this quest, I reserved my GRE date to the following year. Once again, I fought through working full time to study for the entrance exam. As inspired as I was to finally tackle the GRE, another strike occurred and simultaneously I was evicted from my own home by my family. Although my GRE scores were nowhere ideal, my perseverance in finishing that hike on my last day in Ecuador parallels my dedication to becoming a PA student. I took advantage of leaving a third-world country and began to pursue my career in medicine and fulfill my dream. I tenaciously held my GPA while raising my son and working forty hours a week. Not only is my drive focused on my passion for medicine but to inspire my son to demonstrate determination through hardships in his future career. This perseverance and resilience, along with my attention to detail and collaborative nature, will contribute to finishing PA school and earning the privilege of having PA-C at the end of my name.

WITH COMMENTS:

Growing up in rural Peru greatly impacted my family as my mother struggled to single-handedly raise her three children. Before being blessed with the opportunity to relocate to Dallas, TX at the age of 9, we planned to hike a mountain in Peru with our extended family ~~in anticipation of being separated from them for the next 10 years~~. Similarly, this hike compared to organizing my first steps for my career. I strictly focused on my core science subjects in my undergraduate years to ensure success for the possibility of graduate school while working full time. *[This intro provides good personal, background information. I'm not sure that I follow the comparison of the mountain hike to academic planning, but we can see if that is cleared up throughout the rest of the essay. It's okay that PA isn't mentioned yet, but I want to see it included soon.]*

It was a simple march towards my career goals until suddenly, the terrain developed to a steep uphill climb. As I stared down at my positive pregnancy test, I felt the first unsteady footing up this metaphorical mountain in my life. Yet instead of slipping away, I grabbed onto the nearest steady cornerstone and pulled myself up. Deciding to become a single parent at the age of 19 was ultimately the hardest choice I ~~had to~~ endure**d,** but the most profound and proudest moment in my life. *[More helpful personal informa-*

tion. We'll see how these details intertwine with the writer wanting to be in medicine or become a PA. I would likely recommend skipping the mountain metaphor or make it more relevant to PA if possible.] I constructed the objective of never allowing my child to be an excuse for my failures. My family roared in applause as I graduated 7 months pregnant with honors for my associates degree at Fruit Snack College. Furthermore, I persevered in my studies at the University of Popcorn the following fall semester after giving birth to my first-born, Melissa, in July of 2015. *[I love the confidence in the writer's academic success despite a personal challenge. I would love to know what the studies were in and if they were medically relevant to start to incorporate the goal of becoming a PA into the essay more.]*

Fortunately, I mastered the concept of time management skills and academically excelled in my projects by using balance in my routine. I sustained two jobs as a lifeguard and a medical scribe while completing school as a full-time student and ~~being a~~ single parent. An unexpected, yet amazing outcome of my decision to be a medical scribe was learning about the physician assistant (PA) profession. *[This directly is stating how the writer found out about the PA profession. I would like a slightly more clear explanation of how the writer ended up as a medical scribe, but we're getting into the main points of the essay now. A+ for abbreviating correctly.]* While working with a PA, I once witnessed the joint effort of a flawless facilitated admission of a woman in labor to the maternity ward. The PA assured all tests, including pelvic exams, were within normal limits while the physician contacted **the OB/GYN** ~~obgyn~~ department to ensure proper admission. Despite the collaboration between this PA and supervising physician, the course of nature resumed command and conducted the patient dilating from 6 cm to the expulsion of the baby's head in seconds inside the Emergency

Department(ED). *[Yikes! This story is being described well, but could possibly get to the point a little bit quicker.]* I was mesmerized by the partnership and trust between these two providers ~~had~~ to succeed in the delivery of a healthy baby. Witnessing the collaboration between the PA and supervising physician solidified my interest in the medical profession and ultimately ignited my interest towards the PA profession. *[This section is good overall! It shows me the information I'm looking for surrounding PA in a descriptive manner.]*

While scribing for different providers in Central Hospital ED, I ~~was able to~~ work**ed** closely with PAs and truly grasp**ed** their approach to patient evaluation and care. These PAs would thoroughly investigate past medical history, social history, and previous failed treatments of the patient. Even upon discharge, PAs would extensively educate patients by clarifying ED return symptoms, recommend further evaluation with a specialist, and thoroughly instruct them on prescription use. *[These tasks go over the basic tasks PAs can perform, but don't necessarily differentiate PAs from any other healthcare profession. There needs to be a reason specific to PA mentioned as well.]* Additionally, these PAs would insist on prescribing although these medicines could be found over the counter. *[I understand what the writer is trying to say because I work in medicine, but otherwise this reads strangely. By prescribing even though it's OTC, a medication is more likely to be covered by insurance so it's helpful to patients. The way this is written reads as if it's a negative thing though.]* Each PA would demonstrate compassion, sympathy, and most of all time in guaranteeing patient satisfaction and solicitous education. This established my career towards the PA profession as I also yearned in contributing to overall patient satisfaction through the improvement of bedside manner and assuring the patient emotionally. *[These are good goals, but again not specific to being a PA. Some clarification is needed here.]*

After tirelessly researching PA school requirements, I began preparing for my GRE through applying several studying methods to multiply my chances of obtaining my ideal score. Until I experienced a similar downfall to my hike experience in Peru, when I learned of Melissa's half-brother's death. *[Bringing the hike back up now feels strange and out of place and the essay just needs to continue.]* Mentally incapable of continuing this quest, I reserved my GRE date to the following year. Once again, I fought through working full time to study for the entrance exam. As inspired as I was to finally tackle the GRE, another strike occurred and simultaneously I was evicted from my own home by my family. Although my GRE scores were nowhere **near** ideal, my perseverance in finishing that hike on my last day in Ecuador parallels my dedication to becoming a PA student. *[This is a lot of space to devote to a discussion about the GRE when it usually does not carry much weight in the PA school process. I typically don't recommend explaining test scores as long as you meet school requirements. By including life events that had a major effect, it may also make schools question how you would be able to handle PA school if similar issues were to arise. Since this is a conclusion, keep it straightforward and positive.]* I took advantage of leaving a third-world country and began to pursue my career in medicine and fulfill my dream. I tenaciously held my GPA while raising my daughter and working forty hours a week. Not only is my drive focused on my passion for medicine, but to inspire my daughter to demonstrate determination through hardships in his future career. This perseverance and resilience, along with my attention to detail and collaborative nature, will contribute to finishing PA school and earning the privilege of having PA-C at the end of my name. *[Overall, the passion and drive is clear in this essay. There are a few* *areas where clarification of details would be helpful in showing full understanding of the PA profession. There is no mention of the collaborative teamwork approach involved in the job.*

This conclusion does emphasize the strengths of the applicant in an effective manner.]

CHAPTER 18

RESUME REGURGITATION

This essay comes from a waitlisted reapplicant. They consider themselves a non-traditional applicant with lots of stories and service. This essay is 4,784 characters. I don't need to tell you too much about their application because the essay will do it for me!

No statistics from time of application were provided for this example.

ORIGINAL:

I fell in love for the first time when I was seven. The smell of the moss, the taste of the salt around my lips, and the sounds of the thousands of buzzing cicadas consumed me. Many would not appreciate the beauty of that raw nature, but it was special to me. Fishing brought an opportunity to be one with nature and yet to be challenged by its intricacies.

Looking back, I realize what I once loved, and that which gave me peace has transformed. The buzzing of cicadas is now the beeping of a heart rate monitor. And the love, once known in childhood, has metamorphosed into a new devotion. For me, PA school is the advanced commitment.

On January 19, 1996, my mother was driving home when an oncoming vehicle struck her. After eleven days in a coma, she stabilized, permitting her children to see her. In those moments, I saw firsthand that it took a team to heal my mother. Continuing forward, my concerns for justice, benefaction, and aptitude in medicine increased as life continued in a new way for my family. We learned to care for each other as we adjusted to the changes of having a disabled mother.

Then, in high school, I shadowed my first PA, Jordan, where I witnessed service professionally. Our first patient was several weeks pregnant, and due for an ultrasound. Applying the cold gel to the mother's belly, Jordan alleviated the tension stating with a smile, "we only have to do that once." She searched for the baby while listening to the mother's concerns. She was gentle and empathetic as she located the fetal heartbeat, confirming life to the mother and my desire to serve as a PA.

Moving onto college, I enrolled as a pre-PA student. During my final year, I traveled to Ecuador, where I experienced several opportunities to practice communication and understand a new culture. While volunteering at the local hospital, a mother presented with difficulty breastfeeding. She was concerned for her child and unsure of her options. Listening intently, I observed the physician kindly answer the mother's questions and articulate the suggested procedure – a double frenotomy. With the mother's comprehension and approval, he completed the process, demonstrating the importance for every patient to understand the expectations of care clearly. With certitude, I believed that one day, I, too, would embody the healing gifts of gentleness, trust, competence, and adaptability, which I witnessed that day. I was on the path to medicine and yearning for a greater understanding of its mysteries when I embraced another opportunity to serve.

In the summer of 2015, I returned to the US and trained for a bike ride that would cross the nation. Primarily utilizing an online blog and a local radio station as platforms, I raised $9,370.70 for Relay for Life. This effort exceeded my previous philanthropic work, Shave-tober. An event I instituted in 2013 under the Anti-Cancer Foundation to raise awareness for pediatric brain cancer. We raised $2,677 funds and shaved 128 heads, including mine. These endeavors were comprehensive and intense, serving to accentuate my interest in providing service to the cancer community before PA school. Afterward, however, my need for a respite was paramount.

In 2016, I took time away from academia to rest and process life. During this time, I paid off student loans, shadowed a variety of healthcare professionals, reflected on my mother's accident and its ramifications, and confirmed my desire to be a PA as real and constant. Feeling revitalized, I completed senior-level science courses and secured a position with the Dougherty Hospice House, through which I continue to learn the importance of death, compassion, and palliation.

Moreover, at the Doorway Hospice Center, I work alongside diverse, compassionate individuals. They work efficiently and productively without wavering from empathy. Asking our patients and families questions about their mental, physical, emotional, and spiritual needs, they seize the opportunity to connect on deep levels and provide a more integrated, comprehensive solution to the enigma of care. As I continue to prepare for PA school, I deepen my understanding of life, death, and medicine through their examples.

Life, for all of us, is full of ups and downs. With its many mysteries and peak moments of understanding, we grow to better live our lives with new purposes and passions. While the use and love of my life evolve, I press on toward PA school. Just as my mother's accident acted as an initiative for serving, PA school will be a continuation of that desire. My life experiences, medical knowledge, and empathy towards those in difficult situations enables me to meet and honor my patients as they embrace their personal stories. Thus, I am ready to begin my future career as a PA.

WITH COMMENTS:

I fell in love for the first time when I was seven. The smell of the moss, the taste of the salt around my lips, and the sounds of the thousands of buzzing cicadas consumed me. Many would not appreciate the beauty of raw nature, but it was special to me. Fishing brought an opportunity to be one with nature, and yet to be challenged by its intricacies. *[I wasn't sure what the initial descriptors were referring to, but fishing makes sense. I'm now unsure of how that hobby relates to an interest in medicine.]*

Looking back, I realize what I once loved, and that which gave me peace has transformed. The buzzing of cicadas is now the beeping of a heart rate monitor. And the love, once known in childhood, has metamorphosed into a new devotion. For me, **physician assistant** (PA) school is the advanced commitment. *[This feels like a continuation of the intro and this paragraph can likely be combined. The connection between fishing and PA doesn't feel strong enough to have that used as the start to the essay.]*

On January 19, 1996, my mother was driving home when an oncoming vehicle struck her. After eleven days in a coma, she stabilized, permitting her children to see her. In those moments, I saw firsthand that it took a team to heal my mother. Continuing forward, my concerns for justice, benefaction, and aptitude in medicine increased as life continued in a new way for my family. We learned to care for each other as we adjusted to the changes of having a disabled mother. *[It feels like this is indicating how the writer found an interest in medicine after what her mom went through. The date at the beginning is not relevant and would be more helpful if the writer included how old they were at the time of the incident and how their emotions changed throughout this situation. The mentions of "we" need to shift to more personal to the writer.]*

Then, in high school, I shadowed my first PA, Jordan, where I witnessed service professionally. *[This is a big jump from interest in medicine to shadowing a PA. How did the writer find out about PAs and decide to pursue shadowing? We need to be walked through that decision a little more clearly.]* Our first patient was several weeks pregnant, and due for an ultrasound. Applying the cold gel to the mother's belly, Jordan alleviated the tension stating with a smile, "we only have to do that once." *[The dialogue doesn't add anything essential here, and I would recommend taking out.]* She searched for the baby, while listening to the mother's concerns. She was gentle and empathetic as she located the fetal heartbeat, confirming life to the mother and my desire to serve as a PA. *[This shows direct interaction with a PA, but doesn't necessarily tell me how the writer felt about PAs after seeing this exchange with the patient. More detail and personal insight would be helpful.]*

Moving onto college, I enrolled as a pre-PA student. *[That's awesome, but why is this person so drawn to the PA profession? I can't answer that yet.]* During my final year, I traveled to Ecuador, where I experienced several opportunities to practice communication and understand a new culture. While volunteering at the local hospital, a mother presented with difficulty breastfeeding. She was concerned for her child and unsure of her options. Listening intently, I observed the physician kindly answer the mother's questions and articulate the suggested procedure – a double frenotomy. With the mother's comprehension and approval, he completed the process, demonstrating the importance for every patient to understand the expectations of care clearly. With certitude,

I believed that one day, I, too, would embody the healing gifts of gentleness, trust, competence, and adaptability, which I witnessed that day. *[This is a long list of traits. Demonstrating how the writer does them would be more helpful than stating the desire to show them one day.]* I was on the path to medicine and yearning for a greater understanding of its mysteries when I embraced another opportunity to serve. *[Right now, the flow is somewhat disconnected. There isn't a clear connection between paragraphs and topics, although the discussion is in chronological order. It feels like the writer is just reiterating their experiences and not expanding on them in reference to becoming a PA.]*

In the summer of 2015, I returned to the US and trained for a bike ride that would cross the nation. Primarily utilizing an online blog and a local radio station as platforms, I raised $9,370.70 for Relay for Life. This effort exceeded my previous philanthropic work, Shave-tober. An event I instituted in 2013 under the Anti-Cancer Foundation to raise awareness for pediatric brain cancer. We raised $2,677 funds and shaved 128 heads, including mine. These endeavors were comprehensive and intense, serving to accentuate my interest in providing service to the cancer community before PA school. Afterward, however, my need for a respite was paramount. *[These are cool experiences, but why are they in this essay? This takes up a bunch of space, and while it does show a desire for philanthropy, I don't see a clear reason for why this relates to the person wanting to be a PA.]*

In 2016, I took time away from academia to rest and process life. *[Another instance of how providing a year doesn't help me understand when this was without knowing the age of the writer or at what point they were at academically in 2016.]* During this time, I paid off student loans, shadowed a variety of healthcare professionals, reflected on my mother's accident and its ramifications, and confirmed my desire to be a PA as real and constant. Feeling revitalized, I completed senior-level science courses and secured a position with the Dougherty Hospice House, through which I continue to learn the importance of death, compassion, and palliation. *[The information here feels superficial and vague without telling me much more in-depth about how this time really led them to PA more directly.]*

Moreover, at the Doorway Hospice Center, I work alongside diverse, compassionate individuals. They work efficiently and productively without wavering from empathy. Asking our patients and families questions about ~~their~~ mental, physical, emotional, and spiritual needs, they seize the opportunity to connect on deep levels and provide a more integrated, comprehensive solution to the enigma of care. As I continue to prepare for PA school, I deepen my understanding of life, death, and medicine through their examples. *[In this portion, I'm unsure of what exactly the writer's role is in the hospice center. This information would be great in an experience detail section, but isn't very helpful in feeling that the applicant is prepared for PA school based on what's included currently.]*

Life, for all of us, is full of ups and downs. With its many mysteries and peak moments of understanding, we grow to better live our lives with new purposes and passions. *[This is an example of generic, cliche language that isn't specific enough to include in an essay. These metaphorical generalizations use characters without including value.]* While the use and love of my life evolve, I press on toward PA school. Just as my mother's accident acted as an initiative for serving, PA school will be a continuation of that desire. My life experiences, medical knowledge, and empathy towards those in difficult situations enables me to meet and honor my patients as they embrace their personal stories. Thus, I am ready to begin my future career as a PA. *[This essay needs some work. There are personal stories included, which is good, but not enough info to fully say this applicant is ready to take on PA school or become a PA. There is also no discussion of academic success thus far to give me confidence in the applicant's readiness to take on PA school. Most of the information included currently will be covered thoroughly on the application and doesn't need to be repeated directly here.]*

CHAPTER 19

ATHLETE TO PA

We see lots of essays from college athletes. Being in athletics culti-vates great strengths - teamwork, communication, time management - but can be a tough balance between too much focus on the sport and not enough on PA. This essay is 4,952 characters.

No statistics were provided for this example.

ORIGINAL:

As a member of the soccer program at Handprint University, we always made it an emphasis for each of us to know our "Why?". Why are we playing soccer? Why are we at HU? Why do we make the choice to work hard? Why do we sacrifice our time and energy? Personally, I alway knew why I played soccer and made numerous sacrifices to do so. It was because I loved my teammates and I wanted to help them develop as much as I was able to on and off the field. I realized early on that if I did not have fulfilling reasons for doing what I did, I would never reach my ultimate potential. More importantly, I would never be able to help others reach their potential. Since my athletic career has come to an end, the "Why?" that people ask me now is, "Why do you want to be a physician assistant?"

My time as a college athlete taught me valuable lessons that I will call upon throughout my life. I experienced countless obstacles during my career that have refined me into the person I am today. One such obstacle was learning to deal with injury, as most athletes experience at one time or another. Throughout my college soccer and baseball careers I suffered multiple hamstring tears, a broken ankle, a broken tibia, knee issues, and underwent hip surgery after my freshman season. Although my injuries could have been worse, they were debilitating and kept me from doing what I love at the level that I knew I was capable. As a captain of our team it was never easy having to sit on the sideline and watch my team play without me. Being hurt is always mentally and emotionally challenging, but when it affects an entire group of people it makes it much more difficult to cope with. The most frustrating times were when we lost by one or two goals and I knew that I could have made a positive impact on the negative situation. Early on in my college career, I would constantly try to come back earlier than was recommended. I did not want to keep feeling like I was letting my team down and that I was not of value to the program. These thoughts and feelings are not easy burdens to carry on your own. Luckily, I always had great athletic trainers and medical staff that helped me along the way to ease those burdens.

It always seemed that I had very obscure injuries. Before having a hip arthroscopy at 20 years old, I first met with other orthopedists who told me that the injury was simply unfortunate genetics. A year later I had another experience where I was certain that I had broken another bone in my ankle during the middle of a game. As soon as I finished the game, and the adrenaline had worn off, I was unable to walk. After a negative x-ray, I did not know what to think. After a few weeks of rest I was able to play through the consistent pain and finish my sophomore season. Six months later I got an MRI after making no progress in my recovery. The same physician who found my torn labrum just over a year earlier read the MRI. It revealed an occult fracture in my tibia that had been lingering for months. During these instances, and others, I remember always feeling a sense of inexpressible relief that after dwelling in agonizing uncertainty, I was able to get on the right treatment plan and continue doing what I love to do. I owe any success in my athletics to the athletic trainers, physicians, and PAs who provided the care that I needed.

After reevaluating my priorities, I made the decision to end my time as a college athlete with one year of eligibility remaining. I made this decision for a couple of reasons. One was to take more control over my physical and mental well-being. The other reason was that even with how passionate I am about the game of lacrosse, a game that I put 14 years of my life into, I am also very passionate about my choice to pursue a career as a physician assistant. I knew that it was time to truly take it seriously and prepare to the best of my ability.

Although not everybody's situation is the same, most everyone needs their body in prime condition for one reason or another. People rely on medical professionals to keep them going. I chose the path of a physician assistant because I want to develop genuine relationships with the patients that I would have the opportunity to work with. As someone who has been a member and leader on many teams, I know that I have the abilities to be an asset to the medical professional team. Being a PA provides me with the expansive knowledge needed to give back and be that source of relief that so many others have given me. It also provides me the Under not so positive circumstances, I would still get to provide the loving care and support that everybody deserves, but do not always receive. Because my shoulders have carried the same burdens, I want to help lift those burdens off of others as best I can. I believe that my innate desire to help those around me reach their potential will fuel my own potential as a physician assistant. This is my "Why?".

WITH COMMENTS:

As a member of the soccer program at Handprint University, we always made it an emphasis for each of us to know our "Why?" Why are we playing soccer? Why are we at HU? Why do we make the choice to work hard? Why do we sacrifice our time and energy? *[This tells me about the applicant's athletic background straight from the beginning. Teamwork that comes from sports participation is a great personal trait to take into PA school.]* Personally, I alway knew why I played soccer and made numerous sacrifices to do so. It was because I loved my team-mates and I wanted to help them develop ~~as much as I was able to~~ on and off the field. I realized early on that if I did not have fulfilling reasons ~~for doing what I did~~, I would never reach my ultimate potential. More importantly, I would never ~~be able to~~ help others reach their potential. Since my athletic career has come to an end, the "Why?" that people ask me now is, "Why do you want to be a physician assistant **(PA)**?" *[Passion is evident already in this essay, and I appreciate that they are shifting to a discussion surrounding PA quickly.]*

My time as a college athlete taught me valuable lessons ~~that~~ I will call upon throughout my life. I experienced countless obstacles during my career that have refined me into the person I am today. One such obstacle was learning to deal with injury, as most athletes experience at one time or another. Throughout my college soccer and baseball careers I suffered multiple hamstring tears, a broken ankle, a broken tibia, knee issues, and underwent hip surgery after my freshman season. *[Yikes! This shows how personal medical issues have played a role in developing strengths. I'm interested to see if this relates to the writer developing an interest in medicine also.]* Although my injuries could have been worse, they were debilitating and kept me from doing what I love at the level ~~that~~ I knew I was capable. As a captain of our team**,** it was never easy having to sit on the sideline and watch my team play without me. ~~Being hurt is always mentally and emotionally challenging, but when it affects an entire group of people it makes it much more difficult to cope with. The most frustrating times were when we lost by one or two goals and I knew that I could have made a positive impact on the negative situation.~~ *[It's starting to feel like we're dwelling and belaboring this point. Just stating it was disappointing is enough to get that across.]* Early ~~on~~ in my college career, I ~~would~~ constantly ~~try~~ **tried** to come back earlier than ~~was~~ recommended. I did not want to keep feeling like I was letting my team down and that I was not of value to the program. These thoughts and feelings ~~are~~ **were** not easy burdens to carry ~~on your own~~. *[Change anything general to more personal.]* Luckily, I always had great athletic trainers and medical staff that helped me along the way to ease those burdens. *[It's clear that sports played a huge role in the writer's life. They mentioned PA at the beginning, but we need to get into specifics more quickly about how the athletic background relates to an interest in medicine or becoming a PA.]*

It always seemed ~~that~~ I had ~~very~~ obscure injuries. Before having a hip arthroscopy at 20 years old, I first met with other orthopedists who told me ~~that~~ the injury was simply unfortunate genetics. A year later, I had another experience where I was certain ~~that~~ I had broken another bone in my ankle during the middle of a game. As soon as I finished the game, and the adrenaline had worn off, I was unable to walk. After a negative x-ray, ~~I did not know what to think. After~~ **and** a few weeks of rest I was able to play through the consistent pain and finish my sophomore season. Six months later I got an MRI after making no progress in my recovery. The same physician who found my torn labrum just over a year earlier read the MRI. It revealed an occult fracture in my tibia that had been lingering for months. During these instances, and others, I remember ~~always~~ feeling a sense of inexpressible relief that after dwelling in agonizing uncertainty, I was able to get on the right treatment plan and continue doing what I love to do. I owe any success in my athletics to the athletic trainers, physicians, and PAs who provided the care that I needed. *[We're learning a lot about personal injuries, but there aren't any details so far that show us how the writer's personal goals relate to medicine/PA specifically.]*

After reevaluating my priorities, I made the decision to end my time as a college athlete with one year of eligibility remaining. I made this decision for a couple of reasons. One was to take more control over my physical and mental well-being. The other reason was that even with how passionate I am about the game of soccer, a game ~~that~~ I put 14 years of my life into, I am also ~~very~~ passionate about my choice to pursue a career as a **PA** ~~physician assistant~~. I knew ~~that~~ it was time to truly take it seriously and prepare to the best of my ability. *[Everything to this point is surrounding the same topic - the writer's injuries and athletic history. If you were reading this essay without knowing the prompt, what would you think the writer was talking about? We're over halfway through the essay, and I'm still not sure why medicine, why PA, or if there is a strong understanding of the PA profession.]*

Although not everybody's situation is the same, most everyone needs their body in prime condition for one reason or another. People rely on medical professionals to keep them going. I chose the path of a ~~physician assistant~~ **PA** because I want to develop genuine relationships with the patients ~~that~~ I would have the opportunity to work with. As someone who has been a member and leader on many teams, I know ~~that~~ I have the abilities to be an asset to the medical professional team. Being a PA provides me with the expansive knowledge needed to give back and be that source of relief ~~that~~ so many others have given me. It also provides me the Under not so *(?? Make sure to proofread!)* positive circumstances, I would still get to provide the loving care and support ~~that~~ everybody deserves, but do**es** not always receive. *[I'm not really sure what this sentence is trying to indicate, so I would recommend removing.]* Because my shoulders have carried the same burdens, I want to help lift those burdens off of others as best I can. I believe ~~that~~ my innate desire to help those around me reach their potential will fuel my own potential as a **PA** ~~physician assistant~~. ~~This is my "Why?"~~ *[I understand that the writer is trying to tie this in to the beginning of their essay, but it's not a strong way to end. Emphasizing the writer as a PA would be more effective. This conclusion does showcase strengths effectively.]*

I'm missing some essential content from this essay. I don't have any insight into preparations from the writer's experience that would make them ready for PA school or more qualified to be a PA. I don't know if they have any direct interactions with patients other than being one or any volunteer or shadowing experience.

PART 5

BONUS SECTION

CHAPTER 20

EXPERIENCE DETAILS

There are a few questions I get constantly - "How should I do my experience details? Do they matter?" and "How do I make my application stand out?"

Using the Experience Details sections as mini personal statements will make the most of the allowed space and help your essay stand out. The character limit on these sections in CASPA is 600 characters. Since you won't have the space (and shouldn't) expand on each separate experience in your personal statement, you have an opportunity to detail your role and learning points outside of your essay.

I've reviewed a lot of applications. If you've never seen a finalized app, they are typically 25-30 pages long. Each experience is separated by category with information on the location, amount of hours, and then the description you provide. To see an example of this, check out my CASPA videos at www.youtube.com/thepaplatform.

BULLETS VS PARAGRAPHS

Whether to use bullets or paragraphs is the most common concern when it comes to actually writing the experience details section. The CASPA application does not have a specification, leaving it ultimately up to you. In general, schools do not have a preference either. Maintaining consistency with your choice is more important to make your application look nice and easier to follow. I'll give examples in both formats. Even if you choose to write in paragraph form, you don't necessarily need complete sentences. It's okay to be a little brief in this part of your application.

WHAT SHOULD I INCLUDE?

These detail sections are your time to shine and emphasize why your various experiences were impactful in your journey to becoming a PA. The information you include also supports the category you place the experience in, particularly when there is a gray area. For example, if your title is a scribe, but have some duties similar to a medical assistant that fall under patient care experience, you'll need to convince the reader that you have hands-on direct patient exposure. While CASPA has their own definitions of what constitutes each type of experience, the schools hold the ultimate decision about where to categorize your hours.

For that reason, you'll need to lay out your responsibilities in each position, but take it one step further. Also include what you learned from that role. Think about how it will translate into you being more prepared for PA school or a better PA. Brag on yourself and highlight your strengths in these mini personal statements. Try to avoid repetition in stating the same strengths multiple times, but add variety to get the most info in as possible. Head's up - review these sections before heading into an interview just in case you're asked about specifics.

EXAMPLES

Let's go through the bad, good, and great in some of the main categories - patient care experience, volunteering, and shadowing.

―――――――

First up, is patient care experience (PCE). When including these experiences, keep this question in the back of your mind - "Why is this important?" The goal of having PCE is to make certain you want to work in medicine and feel comfortable interacting with patients, not really for learning medicine. That's what PA school is for! Here is a **"bad"** example of a PCE experience details section:

―――――――

Took vitals (BP, pulse, respirations), assisted with activities of daily living and bathing and dressing.

―――――――

Ok. It's way too short and doesn't have nearly enough information. If you have space, I would like to know about the setting and types of patients you were working with. Was it a specific population? This example is a little redundant and doesn't show me anything you gained from being in that position aside from a few skills. Let's move on to a "good" example:

―――――――

In a nursing home setting, I worked as a CNA doing vitals and assisting with activities of daily living, such as bathing, dressing, eating. I talked with my patients and responded to them quickly.

―――――――

This is better with more specifics and hints at a strength without deliberately saying it, but I would still like more details. There's room to add in lessons and strengths with more specifics to show more about what you took out of the role beyond the job description. Here is an example of a "great" description:

In my CNA role in the neuropsych ward of the nursing home, I managed 10-12 patients daily and helped with their ADLs, and monitored vitals. I enjoyed observing my patients improvement by helping with PT exercised and encouraging them through rough days. Learned communication with patient family members in difficult situations.

This tells me so much more! It almost seems like it's referring to a completely different experience than the first example. Does that show you the beauty of how details help? It remains a brief summary highlighting responsibilities, but also includes lessons. This exemplifies how to use abbreviations in experience details. As long as something is commonly known (like ADLs for activities of daily living or PT for physical therapy), feel free to use it. If you're in a niche specialty using abbreviations or tests that aren't widely recognized, you may need to spell it out. For example, I wouldn't include the common abbreviations we use in dermatology because most people outside of the specialty would not be familiar.

Next, let's move on to volunteering examples. What is the point of volunteering? Donating your time demonstrates you care about someone other than yourself and are willing to help. Ideally, your volunteer experience is something you are passionate about and that excitement should come across in your description. You'll notice bullet points to mix it up. Here is a "bad" example based on working in a soup kitchen setting:

- Prepared and served meals
- Helped with clean-up

Yikes! As you can see, multiple issues here. You may be thinking "Surely no one would ever put a description like that!?" Well, you would be surprised how often I've seen it! This description is too short, lacks detail, and is overall not very helpful. The descriptions are valuable, therefore this is wasted potential space. We can make it better:

- Prepared and served meals weekly to homeless populations
- Helped with clean-up while talking with other volunteers

This example provides more detail, which makes it automatically better, however it could still go more in depth. In any experience type discussion, expanding on the type of setting or population you were involved with is helpful in painting a picture for the reader. Going back to one of the first suggestions in this section, there's no mention of the takeaways gained. Consider this more thorough description:

- Prepared and served meals weekly to homeless and primarily Spanish-speaking populations
- Helped with clean-up alongside other volunteers, while sharing our various backgrounds and passion for service
- Assisted in translating when needed and improved communication skills with people from different cultures, as well as empathy through hearing stories from the patrons

The details and specifics in this description give much more information! Of note, this is only around 400 characters, so more room to expand on these points or add in anything notable is available. Just remember, this is valuable real estate so use it to your advantage!

Moving on to shadowing! This section is definitely one of my biggest pet peeves on applications. I rarely see it used correctly. Remember the purpose behind shadowing - to learn about the PA profession and confirm it is the career you want to pursue. The purpose is not necessarily to acquire medical knowledge. Utilizing your experience details is an advantageous way to demonstrate confidence in your understanding of the PA profession, especially when limited by space in the personal statement. This is a shadowing description example is poorly done, but one I see often:

I observed Megan Smith, PA-C. She saw patients for high blood pressure, diabetes, and common colds. I learned how to do wound care and treat heart failure.

The focus isn't where it needs to be, which is on the actual profession of working as a PA, and doesn't tell me much about what the student learned about PAs in that particular setting. It's considerably too short with the given character limit and doesn't emphasize the meaningfulness about this particular experience. Here is a slightly better example:

I shadowed Megan Smith, PA-C, a family medicine PA. I saw her take care of patients and help them with various medical conditions (high blood pressure, diabetes, wound care, colds, flu, heard failure, depression). When she had a question, she asked her collaborating physician.

The additional insight into the setting and type of patients seen during the time with the PA is is an improvement. It highlights some differentiating factors of the PA profession like the relationship with a collaborating physician. Continue to think about "show" instead of "tell." Here is a preferable example:

I shadowed Megan Smith, PA-C, a family medicine PA in her private practice clinic. While observing Megan's interactions with patients, she confidently diagnosed and treated common ailments and chronic conditions, she prescribed medication and performed basic procedures like ear irrigation and wound care. I saw how Megan treated patients autonomously, and consulted with her collaborating physician on complex cases when needed. This experience encourages me to seek a similar relationship in the future, and inspires me towards my goal of becoming a PA.

This example includes everything the reader is looking for! It sums up observations from that setting succinctly without too much detail about specific conditions. In reading these descriptions, this last one emphasizes how knowledgeable the PA was, but also the collaborative approach of the PA profession. At 557 characters, there is space to discuss both what you witnessed and gained from any experience.

STRENGTHS/LESSONS TO CONSIDER

Here are suggestions you may want to highlight in some experiences when relevant:

- Communication - with patients, patient family members, co-workers, other medical professionals, supervisors
- Conflict resolution
- Empathy
- Compassion with patients
- Handling difficult patients - This could be a frustrated patient or a case that takes an emotional toll on you.
- Passion for whatever you're involved in - patient care, volunteering

SKILLS TO INCLUDE

Think about including and highlighting specific skills that could potentially make you stand out as an applicant and will ultimately make you a superior student.

- Taking blood pressure and other vital signs
- Phlebotomy
- Administering injections
- Familiarity with a certain specialty
- Casting/splinting
- Administrative work - answering phones, communicating with insurance companies, prior authorizations, billing

---

If you need professional help editing your experience details, visit thePAplatform.com for information on editing services.

CHAPTER 21

SUPPLEMENTAL ESSAYS

Beyond your personal statement, many schools require additional essays to gain insight about each applicant. These will be school specific and allow you to expand on the points you couldn't fully explain in your main essay. These responses are important because the schools have chosen these prompts for specific reasons. They will focus on what is important and relevant to them as a program, coincidentally this gives you additional insight about the school's mission. Check program websites to verify if a supplemental application is required. In some cases, supplementals are only sent out after your universal application is received through CASPA or only to certain candidates.

Prepare adequate time to write your supplemental essays. Keep in mind, number of essays and length requirements vary greatly between schools. I've seen responses that only allow for 250 characters, and others with 5 separate one page essays! Take that into account when planning how many programs you'll apply to. It can be tempting to spread a wide net to 25+ schools, but you likely won't have sufficient time to complete all essays efficiently. As a reapplicant, consider editing your supplementals to ensure they reflect improvements. Also, double check the prompts and requirements because schools may amend them between cycles.

The good news about these essays is there does seem to be consistency in the topics covered between programs - addressing their mission, expanding on experience or grades, and filling in application gaps. That's beneficial for you as an applicant because you can repurpose responses. Change anything school specific and make certain the details are applicable to the correct program.

Since these are school specific, use the program website as your guide in responding. Attempt to apply specific wording from the mission statement, technical standards, and incorporate program objectives in your writing. I also recommend utilizing wording from the prompt into your responses as well. This tactic helps the programs feel confident that you've answered thoroughly.

LOGISTICS

Depending on the character limit, using abbreviations will be more acceptable for supplemental essays. If you already used an abbreviation in a different supplemental or your personal statement, feel free to repeat it without spelling out the long form version.

If your supplemental doesn't have a specific length limit, or some crazy amount like 10,000 characters, continue to be mindful of your reader's time. No longer than one page if possible because it really shouldn't take much more to fully get your point across. Utilize the prompts as a guide to ensure everything included in your response answers the question directly.

This should go without saying, but nothing should be directly copied from your personal statement. Expand on the points you've made there, but in a completely different way. Pay attention to how the prompts are worded. If it asks for a list, your response should be a list! Be direct in how you respond to make the most of the space available.

EXAMPLE PROMPTS

Here are just a few examples of different supplemental prompts directly from applications.

- With over 200 accredited PA programs in the U.S., why have you chosen to apply to XYZ University?
- Describe what contribution you can make to the PA profession and to XYZ's PA program.
- If you are a re-applicant, to XYZ, what was the final outcome of your prior application(s) and what changes, if any, have you made which should result in a different outcome?
- What are the personal attributes you possess and/or the activities in which you've been involved which demonstrate your commitment to our mission statement?
- How do you envision fulfilling our mission as a graduate of this program?
- Please tell us about an experience you've had participating in service to the community and how this experience has enhanced your preparation for the physician assistant profession.
- What challenges will your education in Public Health enable you to address in providing primary care to underserved populations?
- Does your academic record accurately reflect who you are as a student? Please explain. Do you feel your academic record accurately reflects how you will perform in a PA Program?

For professional help with editing your supplemental essays, check out thePAplatform.com.

CHAPTER 22

INTERVIEW ESSAYS

This chapter is a (slightly modified) sneak preview from the Physician Assistant School Interview Guide. Once you submit your application and begin interview preparation, check it out on Amazon or thepaplatform.com/book.

———

This chapter will be short and sweet! Some schools ask you to write an essay during the interview. It may be one essay, or a few short answer questions, but typically nothing too intense. Try not to stress about this possibility too much! Writing a short, timed essay should not add to your nerves significantly. If you adequately prepared for your interview and wrote your own personal statement, you should be fine.

Schools have a few motives for asking you to write an essay. The first is to verify you as the author of your personal statement and see if the prose aligns. Your personal statement will be much more detailed and polished than the essay you write during the interview, but a large discrepancy in writing style would be apparent. Programs are aware of companies that write entire essays for students, which is highly unethical.

Another objective is to ensure fluency in English. If English is not your first language, this is a chance to demonstrate high quality writing skills in English. PAs are required to write medical notes, which need to be easily understood by other individuals who review the information in a patient's chart.

When writing an essay, demonstrate the ability to form an opinion. The capability to organize your thoughts on a subject in a concise way and convey them on paper is your primary goal. The time limit is usually short, typically 30 minutes, or you'll have the entire day to complete your response during downtime.

When it was time for my essay portion during interviews, I had prepared a strategy. I wasn't going to attempt a literary piece of art. I simply wanted to get my answer down as quickly as possible knowing there could be a limited amount of time. At my interview, we were given 30 minutes at the end of the day to complete the essay portion. Some interviews provide the prompt at the beginning of the day, leaving you to work on writing during downtime, and you turn it in before leaving.

I resorted to 5th grade essay writing techniques. Just the basics!

- An introduction laying out what I was planning to discuss
- 3 body paragraphs with their own main point and supporting details
- A short conclusion summarizing the entire essay

Nothing too crazy happening in my PA interview essays! Space may be limited, and there's only so much one can say in 1-2 pages. Keep in mind that expectations are not extravagant for this essay, and the weight of your actual face to face interview is much more influential.

The essay could be a specific topic, or just a traditional interview question, for example "Why do you want to be a PA?" It could also be an ethical question. You may be asked to read an article and discuss your opinions about the medical or ethical issue presented. Also, prepare for off the wall questions, such as "If you could have any super power, what would it be and why?" Prior to your interview, I suggest practice writing a 1-page response to any typical interview questions, the prompts below, or from the previous supplemental essay chapter.

Suggested prompts:

- Why did you choose to apply to our program?
- Explain what you think is the biggest challenge facing physician assistants, and how you plan to address it as a PA.
- What are your 3 biggest strengths?
- What qualities are found in a successful PA?

How to practice:

- Choose a prompt to practice your interview essay skills.
- Set a timer for 30 minutes.
- Sit down with paper and pen, and write out your response.
- Ask friends or family to evaluate your essay, or post in the PA Platform forum at https://www.thepaplatform.com/physicianassistantforum

SO WHAT'S NEXT?

Now that you've completed the book, I hope you have a fully written essay, or at least feel prepared to start. To stay up to date on current events in the PA field, join our monthly newsletter - www. thepaplatform.com/newsletter

If you enjoyed the book, and feel you gained valuable knowledge, I would be forever grateful for an Amazon review to help other PA hopefuls know what to expect.

Bulk orders of the book are available for Pre-PA Clubs at a discounted rate. You can go to www.thepaplatform.com/psbook for more information.

If you've finished your essay, but need help with editing, head to www.thepaplatform.com for personalized guidance. The PA Platform exclusively uses physician assistants for editing, and we provide feedback on content, flow, and grammar to make sure your essay is ready for submission. Use the code FUTUREPA for a discount on your editing service.

Don't forget the golden rule: The essay gets the interview, and the interview gets you accepted. Once you get that interview invite, check out The PA School Interview Guide for interview tips. As always, email The PA Platform with any questions at info@thepaplatform.com.

- Savanna

Need more help?

Personal Statement Editing
is available at
ThePAPlatform.com

Let one of our experienced PAs help polish your essay and make it ready for submission. With editing of content, grammar, and flow, we'll make sure you feel confident with the final product.

Discount Code:
FUTUREPA

+ Supplemental Essays, Experience Details, etc.

RESOURCES

The PA Platform - The best information for hopeful pre-PA students on the path to becoming physician assistants - thepaplatform.com

You'll find blog posts, webinars, videos, and free downloads to help you feel prepared during this journey to PA school. Use the code PSBOOK for a discount on any service or product from The PA Platform or on prepacourses.com.

Follow on social media for the most recent announcements:

- Instagram: @thePAplatform
- Facebook: http://www.facebook.com/thePAplatform
- Youtube: http://www.youtube.com/thePAplatform
- Pinterest: http://www.pinterest.com/thePAplatform
- Twitter: http://www.twitter.com/thePAplatform
- TikTok: @physicianassistant

THE PRE-PA CLUB PODCAST

For weekly podcast episodes, subscribe to The Pre-PA Club Podcast on iTunes, or visit http://www.thepaplatform.com/podcast to access all episodes. We frequently interview PAs and PA students, and you can leave a voicemail question for the podcast.

THE PRE-PA CLUB FACEBOOK GROUP

The PA Platform runs a Facebook group exclusive to Pre-PA students called "The Pre-PA Club." By joining, you can ask questions and get feedback from practicing PAs and your peers.

GET SOME FREE STUFF!

To thank you for purchasing my book, I want to give you a free video course! We'll walk through an essay step-by-step. Visit the link below and use code PSBOOK to get the Personal Statement Workshop + Live Editing now!

HTTP://WWW.PREPACOURSES.COM

Be sure to check out our other courses at www.prepacourses.com including our past conferences!

Services on The PA Platform

Mock Interview - Once you've nailed your personal statement, you need to rock the interview. Doing a mock interview will prepare you for the type of questions that will be asked and help calm your nerves. What's included: 60 minutes total with a practicing PA, personalized interview experience based on your application, tips and techniques for your specific interview, 20-30 minutes of questions, feedback following Q&A session.

Pre-PA Assessment - Send your credentials and we'll evaluate your strength as a candidate and help you come up with a strategy to become an even more competitive applicant. Great for high school students, undergraduate students, any first-time applicant or reapplicants! What's included: A pre-assessment of your current GPA and experience by a practicing PA, CASPA GPA prediction and calculator, a written summary and plan, 20 minute video session with a Pre-PA coach

Supplemental Essay Review - Once your initial application is complete, you may have additional supplemental applications to work on. This is your chance to tell the admissions committee even more about yourself and why you should be in their program.

www.thepaplatform.com/services-1

PSBOOK FOR 10% OFF

After submitting your application for physician assistant school, the interview is next. Does the thought of a face-to-face encounter that will decide your future scare you? Are you worried about saying the "right" thing? You're not alone. In Physician Assistant School Interview Guide, Savanna Perry, PA-C walks you through the steps of taking control of your interview and using your personal accomplishments to impress your interviewers.

In these pages, you'll learn how to:

Prepare for your specific PA school interview by familiarizing yourself with various interview techniques

Stand above the crowd with the knowledge to understand the motives behind the questions

Develop thoughtful, mature answers to commonly asked questions

Gain the confidence needed to secure your spot in a PA program

This interview is your chance to impress your future alma mater and move one step closer to becoming a PA. This book is the key to help you reach your goal.

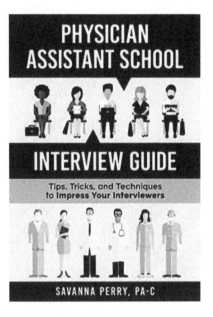

Your interview earns you an acceptance to PA school.

Rock your interview.

Perfect your interviewing skills with a mock interview conducted by one of our Pre-PA Coaches,.

www.ThePAPlatform.com/mock-interview

PSBOOK FOR 10% OFF

PART 6

NOTES

Made in USA - Kendallville, IN
39934_9781732076013
12.22.2021 1808